KIDNEY- FRIENDLY VEGETARIAN COOKBOOK FOR BEGINNERS

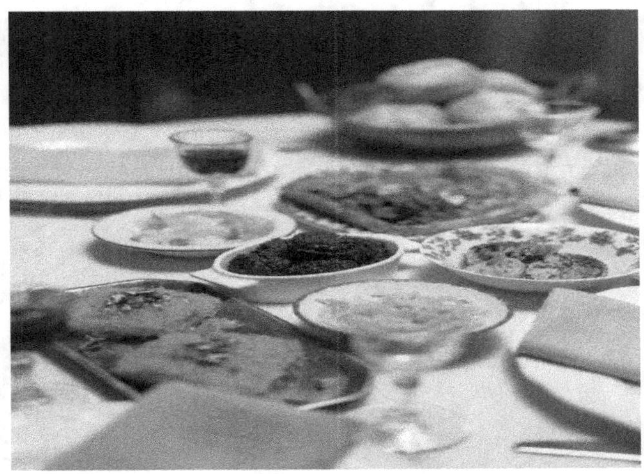

NOURISHING VEGETARIAN RECIPES FOR KIDNEY WELLNESS

ANNIE ANDERSON

Table of Contents

• 1/2 cup unsweetened almond milk (low in potassium) 102

• 1/4 cup fresh blueberries (antioxidant-rich) 102

• 1/4 cup fresh strawberries, sliced (low in potassium) 102

• 1 tablespoon chia seeds (omega-3 fatty acids) 102

• 1 tablespoon chopped almonds (low in potassium, high in healthy fats) 102

• 1/2 teaspoon cinnamon (adds flavor without sodium) 102

• 1/2 teaspoon vanilla extract (adds sweetness without added sugars) 102

• Optional: 1 teaspoon honey or maple syrup (use sparingly for sweetness) 102

Instructions: 102

Combine Dry Ingredients: 102

1. In a mason jar or airtight container, mix the old-fashioned oats, chia seeds, chopped almonds, and cinnamon. These ingredients provide a balance of fiber, healthy fats, and essential nutrients without overloading on phosphorus or potassium. 103

Add Wet Ingredients: 103

2. Add vanilla essence and unsweetened almond milk. Almond milk is a kidney-friendly alternative to dairy, and vanilla extract adds natural sweetness without resorting to high-sugar options. 103

Incorporate Berries: 103

3. Gently fold in the fresh blueberries and sliced strawberries. Berries are rich in

antioxidants, vitamins, and fiber, making
them excellent choices for kidney health
without contributing excessive potassium.

4. Mix all ingredients thoroughly, ensuring
an even distribution of flavors. Seal the
container and refrigerate overnight. This
enables the flavors to combine and the oats

5. Stir well the next morning with the oats. If
desired, drizzle a small amount of honey or
maple syrup for sweetness. However, be
mindful of added sugars, and use these

6. Enhance the visual appeal and nutritional
content by topping the oats with a few extra
fresh berries. This provides a burst of flavor

7. Savour the kidney-friendly overnight oats
with berries mindfully, appreciating the
combination of textures and flavors. This
breakfast option offers a balance of
essential nutrients while adhering to the
dietary considerations necessary for kidney

By focusing on low-phosphorus and
low-potassium ingredients, incorporating
healthy fats from almonds and chia seeds,
and leveraging the antioxidant benefits of
berries, this comprehensive overnight oats

One of the primary functions of the kidneys is to filter waste products and toxins from the bloodstream, forming urine as a means of excretion. Adequate water intake is crucial for this filtration process. When the body is well-hydrated, the blood volume remains stable, allowing the kidneys to effectively remove waste and maintain a proper balance of electrolytes. This optimal blood volume ensures that the kidneys can perform their filtration duties without unnecessary strain. 152

Furthermore, water plays a key role in preventing the formation of kidney stones. Kidney stones are crystallized deposits that can develop when the urine becomes too concentrated, leading to the precipitation of minerals. Insufficient water intake contributes to the concentration of urine, making it more conducive to stone formation. By drinking an ample amount of water, individuals dilute their urine, reducing the risk of mineral crystallization and the subsequent development of kidney stones. This preventive aspect underscores the importance of water in preserving kidney health. 153

Proper hydration is also essential for preventing urinary tract infections (UTIs), which can adversely affect kidney function. The urinary tract, including the bladder and urethra, is susceptible to bacterial infections. Water helps flush out bacteria from the urinary system, reducing the likelihood of infection. Inadequate water intake can lead to stagnant urine, providing an environment conducive to bacterial growth. A well-hydrated body, on the other hand, promotes the continual flushing of bacteria, minimizing the risk of UTIs and safeguarding the kidneys from potential harm. 154

Beyond its role in specific kidney-related conditions, water contributes to overall metabolic processes that indirectly impact renal wellness. Hydration supports digestion, nutrient absorption, and the transportation of essential substances throughout the body. The kidneys rely on these systemic processes to receive nutrients and oxygen for their own well-being. Thus, maintaining an adequate water balance ensures that the kidneys receive the necessary resources to function optimally.   155

In addition to preventing kidney stones and urinary tract infections, water aids in the regulation of blood pressure. The kidneys play a pivotal role in blood pressure regulation by adjusting the volume of blood and the concentration of electrolytes. When the body is adequately hydrated, blood volume remains stable, allowing the kidneys to maintain optimal blood pressure. Proper blood pressure is crucial for preserving the structural integrity of the kidneys and preventing long-term damage associated with hypertension.   156

In conclusion, the importance of water in relation to kidney wellness cannot be overstated. From facilitating the filtration of waste products to preventing the formation of kidney stones and urinary tract infections, water is a cornerstone of renal health. Its impact extends beyond the kidneys, influencing overall bodily functions that are intricately connected to renal well-being. As we recognize the vital role water plays in sustaining life, we concurrently acknowledge its indispensable role in maintaining the health and functionality of one of the body's most vital organs—the kidneys. 157

Navigating restaurant menus with kidney wellness in mind involves strategic choices that prioritize low-potassium, low-phosphorus, and low-sodium options. By understanding your dietary restrictions and communicating them to restaurant staff, you can enjoy a satisfying and kidney-friendly dining experience. Making informed decisions about what goes on your plate contributes to the overall well-being of your kidneys and supports a healthier lifestyle.   190

Maintaining kidney wellness is crucial for overall health, and dietary choices play a pivotal role in supporting kidney function. Communicating dietary needs in the context of kidney wellness involves understanding the specific dietary restrictions and recommendations that can help manage conditions such as chronic kidney disease (CKD). Individuals with kidney issues must work closely with healthcare professionals, including dietitians and nephrologists, to develop a personalized dietary plan tailored to their needs.   191

Firstly, it's essential to grasp the significance of dietary adjustments in promoting kidney health. The kidneys play a vital role in filtering waste and excess fluids from the blood, and when they are compromised, certain dietary modifications become imperative. Patients with CKD, for instance, may need to monitor their protein intake, as excessive protein can strain the kidneys. Communicating this aspect involves educating individuals on choosing high-quality protein sources, such as lean meats, poultry, fish, and plant-based options like legumes. 192

Sodium, another critical element, requires meticulous attention. High sodium levels can contribute to fluid retention and elevated blood pressure, both detrimental to kidney function. Communicating the need to limit sodium intake involves educating individuals about hidden sources of sodium in processed foods and encouraging the use of herbs and spices for flavoring instead. Emphasizing the importance of reading food labels becomes crucial for making informed choices. 193

Fluid management is equally vital in kidney wellness. Individuals may need to adjust their fluid intake based on their specific kidney condition. Communicating this involves conveying the importance of staying hydrated while being mindful of excessive fluid intake, which can strain the kidneys. Encouraging the use of thirst as a guide for fluid consumption can be an effective way to communicate this aspect of kidney-friendly nutrition. 194

Phosphorus and potassium are minerals that also demand attention in kidney wellness. High levels of these minerals can disrupt the balance in the body and pose challenges for individuals with compromised kidney function. Communicating the need to monitor phosphorus involves educating individuals about its presence in various foods, especially processed and fast foods. Similarly, guiding individuals on managing potassium intake includes highlighting low-potassium food choices and the importance of portion control. 195

In communicating dietary needs for kidney wellness, collaboration with healthcare professionals is paramount. Dietitians play a crucial role in translating medical recommendations into practical dietary advice. Communicating with a dietitian allows individuals to receive personalized guidance based on their specific health status, preferences, and cultural considerations. Dietitians can help create meal plans that align with dietary restrictions, ensuring optimal nutrition while safeguarding kidney health. 196

Moreover, incorporating a multidisciplinary approach involving nephrologists further enhances communication about dietary needs. Nephrologists can provide insights into the progression of kidney disease and collaborate with dietitians to fine-tune dietary recommendations accordingly. This collaborative effort reinforces the importance of a holistic approach to kidney wellness. 197

Family and community support are integral aspects of effective communication

regarding dietary needs for kidney wellness.
Educating family members and close friends
about the dietary restrictions and
preferences of individuals with kidney
issues fosters a supportive environment.
This involves dispelling misconceptions and
promoting awareness to ensure that social
gatherings and shared meals align with
kidney-friendly choices.   198

In conclusion, communicating dietary needs
in relation to kidney wellness requires a
comprehensive understanding of the
intricacies involved in managing conditions
like CKD. From protein intake to sodium
restriction and fluid management, conveying
these aspects involves education,
collaboration with healthcare professionals,
and fostering a supportive community. By
integrating these elements, individuals can
navigate their dietary journey with a focus
on kidney health, contributing to an overall
enhanced quality of life.   199

Vegetarianism has gained popularity for its
perceived health benefits, environmental
considerations, and ethical reasons.
However, when it comes to kidney wellness,
there are several myths surrounding

vegetarian protein sources that need clarification. Understanding these myths is crucial for individuals, as misinformation may lead to dietary choices that could impact kidney health.   212

One common myth is that plant-based proteins lack completeness, meaning they do not provide all essential amino acids necessary for the body. While it is true that some plant-based proteins may be deficient in one or more amino acids, a well-balanced vegetarian diet can easily overcome this limitation. Combining various plant-based protein sources, such as legumes, grains, nuts, and seeds, ensures a diverse amino acid profile, providing the body with the essential building blocks it needs.   213

Another misconception is that plant-based proteins are insufficient in quantity, making it challenging to meet daily protein requirements. In reality, many plant-based foods are rich in protein, and with proper planning, individuals can easily achieve their protein needs through a vegetarian diet. Lentils, chickpeas, tofu, quinoa, and edamame are just a few examples of protein-packed plant foods that can contribute significantly to daily protein intake.   214

A prevailing myth suggests that plant-based proteins are harder to digest compared to animal proteins. While it is true that some individuals may experience gas or bloating initially when incorporating more plant-based foods, these symptoms often subside as the digestive system adjusts.

Additionally, proper cooking methods, such as soaking, sprouting, or fermenting, can enhance the digestibility of plant-based proteins.   215

There is a misconception that vegetarian diets lead to nutrient deficiencies, particularly in essential minerals like iron and calcium. In the context of kidney wellness, it's important to note that excessive consumption of animal proteins can burden the kidneys and potentially lead to kidney issues. Plant-based diets, when properly planned, can provide ample nutrients, including iron and calcium, without the negative impact on kidney health associated with high animal protein intake. 216

Some individuals believe that vegetarian diets lack protein variety, leading to monotony and potential nutritional deficiencies. However, the plant kingdom offers a wide array of protein sources, each with its unique set of nutrients and flavors. From the vast selection of legumes, grains, nuts, seeds, and plant-based protein products, individuals can create diverse and satisfying meals that cater to their protein needs.   217

Concerns about inadequate protein quality in plant-based diets often stem from misconceptions about protein digestibility and absorption. While plant-based proteins may have slightly lower bioavailability than animal proteins, this doesn't mean they are inadequate. Including a variety of protein sources and complementing them with other

Nutritionists play a crucial role in guiding individuals toward a kidney-friendly vegetarian diet, offering valuable insights that promote renal health while adhering to plant-based principles. As more people embrace vegetarianism for various reasons, including ethical, environmental, and health considerations, understanding how to maintain kidney wellness within this dietary framework becomes essential. Here are comprehensive insights from nutritionists on crafting a kidney-friendly vegetarian diet. 229

Balanced Plant-Based Proteins: 229

1. Nutritionists emphasize the importance of incorporating a variety of plant-based proteins to ensure a comprehensive amino acid profile. Legumes, such as lentils, chickpeas, and beans, are excellent sources of protein, and when combined with whole grains, nuts, and seeds, they form a complete protein spectrum. Ensuring an adequate intake of protein is essential for overall health and muscle function, especially for individuals with kidney concerns. 230

Mindful Phosphorus Management: 230

2. Nutritionists highlight the significance of managing phosphorus intake, as excessive levels can be detrimental to kidney health. While plant-based foods generally contain less absorbable phosphorus than animal products, some high-phosphorus plant foods, such as nuts and seeds, should be consumed in moderation. Cooking techniques like leaching and soaking can help reduce phosphorus content in certain foods, supporting kidney wellness. 230

Calcium-Rich Plant Sources: 230

3. Maintaining optimal calcium levels is crucial

for bone health, and nutritionists advise individuals to explore plant-based calcium sources. Dark leafy greens like kale and bok choy, fortified plant milks, and tofu made with calcium sulfate are excellent alternatives. Ensuring an adequate intake of calcium while being mindful of phosphorus levels contributes to a balanced kidney-friendly vegetarian diet. 231

Strategic Potassium Control: 231

4. Nutritionists stress the importance of managing potassium levels, especially for individuals with kidney issues. While many plant-based foods are high in potassium, including fruits, vegetables, and legumes, portion control and strategic food choices can help regulate potassium intake. Cooking methods, such as boiling or leaching, can further assist in reducing potassium content in certain foods.   232

Fluid Balance and Hydration: 232

5. Nutritionists emphasize the significance of maintaining proper fluid balance for kidney health. Adequate hydration supports kidney function and helps flush out waste products. Water, herbal teas, and low-sugar beverages are recommended choices. Monitoring fluid intake becomes essential, especially for individuals with kidney concerns who may need to limit fluid consumption based on their specific health requirements.   232

Individualized Nutrient Needs: 232

6. Nutritionists underscore the importance of individualized nutrition plans tailored to specific health needs and preferences. Each person's

nutritional requirements vary, and factors such as age, gender, activity level, and overall health should be considered. Consulting with a registered dietitian allows individuals to receive personalized guidance on crafting a kidney-friendly vegetarian diet that aligns with their unique nutritional needs.   233

Vitamin D and Sun Exposure: 233

7. Ensuring adequate vitamin D levels is crucial for kidney health, as it plays a role in calcium absorption. Nutritionists recommend incorporating vitamin D-rich foods like fortified plant milks and cereals or considering vitamin D supplements if necessary. Additionally, moderate sun exposure contributes to natural vitamin D synthesis, supporting overall bone and kidney wellness.   234

Mindful Sodium Consumption: 234

8. Nutritionists emphasize the importance of mindful sodium control, as excessive salt intake can contribute to hypertension and negatively impact kidney function. Choosing fresh, whole foods and using herbs and spices for flavoring instead of salt are practical strategies. Reading food labels helps identify hidden sources of sodium in processed and packaged vegetarian products.   234

Gradual Dietary Changes: 234

9. Nutritionists advocate for gradual dietary changes, especially for those transitioning to a vegetarian lifestyle. Slowly introducing new foods and experimenting with different recipes allows individuals to adapt to the dietary shift while monitoring how their bodies respond. This approach promotes long-term adherence to a

10. Nutritionists emphasize the importance of regular monitoring of kidney function through medical check-ups and blood tests. Adjustments to the diet may be necessary based on individual health changes and evolving nutritional needs. Nutritionists work collaboratively with healthcare providers to ensure that dietary recommendations align with overall health goals. 235

In conclusion, insights from nutritionists play a pivotal role in guiding individuals toward a kidney-friendly vegetarian diet. By focusing on balanced plant-based proteins, strategic nutrient management, individualized nutrition plans, and gradual dietary changes, individuals can embrace a vegetarian lifestyle while supporting optimal kidney health. Nutritionists provide valuable expertise in navigating the complexities of dietary choices, empowering individuals to make informed decisions that promote both their vegetarian principles and renal wellness. 236

*1. Q: Can I get enough protein from a vegetarian diet to support kidney health? 236

A: Absolutely. While animal products are common protein sources, a well-planned vegetarian diet can provide ample protein. Legumes, tofu, tempeh, nuts, and seeds are rich in protein and can be combined to ensure a complete amino acid profile, supporting kidney health without

A: Yes. Plant-based proteins offer numerous health benefits and can be favorable for kidney health. They tend to be lower in phosphorus, which is crucial for those with kidney concerns. Legumes, grains, and plant-based protein products can serve as excellent alternatives to animal proteins while supporting overall well-being.

A: Focus on moderation and mindful choices. While some plant foods contain phosphorus, it's about balancing the intake. Limit high-phosphorus foods like nuts and seeds, and consider cooking methods that reduce phosphorus, such as leaching or boiling vegetables. Regular monitoring and consulting with a dietitian can help manage phosphorus levels effectively.

A: Yes, in moderation. Dairy products are good sources of calcium, but they can be high in phosphorus. Opt for lower-phosphorus dairy options or explore plant-based alternatives like almond or rice milk fortified with calcium. Again, moderation is key to strike the right balance.

A: Absolutely. Dark leafy greens like kale and bok choy, fortified plant milks, and tofu made with calcium sulfate are excellent sources of plant-based calcium. Including these foods in your diet ensures that you meet your calcium needs without compromising kidney health. 239

A: Be mindful of high-potassium foods like bananas, oranges, and potatoes. Portion control is essential, and cooking techniques like boiling or leaching can help reduce potassium content. Including a variety of fruits and vegetables while monitoring portions allows you to enjoy a diverse diet without exceeding potassium limits. 240

A: Yes, with proper planning. A well-structured vegetarian diet can be suitable for kidney health. It involves choosing the right mix of plant-based proteins, managing phosphorus and potassium levels, and staying hydrated. Consulting with a dietitian ensures that dietary choices align with individual health needs. 240

A: Certainly. Opt for kidney-friendly snacks like air-popped popcorn, raw vegetables with hummus, or a small serving of mixed nuts. Reading labels to identify hidden

phosphorus or sodium in packaged snacks
is essential. Balancing taste and nutrition is
achievable with mindful snack choices.   241

9. Q: How can I add flavor to my meals
without using too much salt?   241

A: Get creative with herbs, spices, and
citrus flavors. Fresh herbs like basil,
cilantro, and mint, along with spices such as
cumin, coriander, and turmeric, can add
depth and flavor to your dishes without
relying on excessive salt. Experimenting
with different combinations enhances the
taste of kidney-friendly meals.   241

10. Q: Can I still enjoy international
cuisines on a kidney-friendly vegetarian
diet?   241

A: Absolutely. Many international cuisines
offer a variety of plant-based options. For
example, Mediterranean cuisine includes
dishes like lentil soups and grilled
vegetables, and Asian cuisine often features
tofu and vegetable stir-fries. Exploring
diverse cuisines ensures that you can enjoy
flavorful meals while adhering to
kidney-friendly guidelines.   242

11. Q: How do I ensure I'm getting
enough vitamins and minerals on a
vegetarian diet?   242

A: Variety is key. Including a diverse range
of fruits, vegetables, whole grains, nuts, and
seeds ensures you receive a spectrum of
essential nutrients. If there are concerns
about specific nutrients, consulting with a
dietitian can help create a personalized plan
to address individual nutritional needs.   242

layering the layers on. colorful layers not only look appealing but also provide a variety of flavors and textures.	248

Drizzle with Honey or Maple Syrup (Optional):	248

5. If you desire a touch of sweetness, drizzle a small amount of honey or maple syrup over the top. Keep in mind that excessive sugar intake should be avoided, so use this option sparingly or skip it altogether. The natural sweetness from the berries may be sufficient to satisfy your taste buds.	248

Garnish with Fresh Mint:	248

6. Add a finishing touch to your berry parfait by garnishing it with fresh mint leaves. Not only does mint enhance the visual appeal, but it also contributes a refreshing flavor that complements the sweetness of the berries.	249

Effect on the Body:	249

Rich in Antioxidants:	249

1. Berries are packed with antioxidants, such as anthocyanins and vitamin C, which help combat oxidative stress and inflammation. These properties are beneficial for overall health and may contribute to kidney wellness.	249

Protein and Calcium for Kidney Health:	249

2. Greek yogurt serves as an excellent source of protein and calcium. Protein is essential for muscle function, and calcium is crucial for bone health. Incorporating these nutrients in a kidney-friendly dessert

excess core helps make room for the delicious stuffing. 254

3. Mix the Filling: In a bowl, combine cinnamon, sweetener, and a splash of vanilla extract. Adjust the sweetness according to your taste and dietary requirements. If you're adding nuts, mix them into the cinnamon-sweetener mixture. 254

4. Stuff the Apples: Spoon the cinnamon-sweetener mixture into the well of each apple. Ensure an even distribution of the filling for consistent flavor. 255

5. Top with Butter or Margarine: Place a small amount of kidney-friendly butter or margarine on top of each stuffed apple. This adds a rich, buttery flavor while keeping saturated fat levels in check. 255

6. Bake to Perfection: Arrange the stuffed apples in a baking dish and bake in the preheated oven for approximately 25-30 minutes or until the apples are tender. Baking time may vary based on the size and variety of apples, so keep an eye on them. 255

7. Serve Warm: Once baked, let the apples cool slightly before serving. The warmth of the baked apples, combined with the aromatic cinnamon, creates a comforting and inviting dessert. 255

This kidney-friendly baked apple with cinnamon dessert is a wholesome treat that balances sweetness and nutrition. It provides a satisfying alternative to traditional desserts that may be high in

INTRODUCTION

In a world where dietary choices play a pivotal role in our well-being, embracing a kidney-friendly vegetarian lifestyle is a compassionate journey towards optimal health. For those navigating the intricate landscape of renal wellness, a reliable guide is indispensable. Enter the "Harmony in Greens: A Kidney-Friendly Vegetarian Cookbook for Beginners," a culinary compass designed to transform your kitchen into a sanctuary of nourishment.

As the demand for kidney-friendly dietary resources rises, this cookbook emerges as a beacon for individuals seeking not only delectable plant-based recipes but also a profound understanding of how to support kidney health. The term 'vegetarian' often conjures images of vibrant produce and innovative dishes, but this cookbook goes beyond the surface, delving into the intricacies of crafting meals that are not only delicious but also tailored to nurture kidney function.

Embarking on a renal-friendly vegetarian journey can be intimidating, especially for beginners. "Harmony in Greens" takes this challenge head-on, offering a comprehensive introduction that demystifies the complexities of kidney-friendly nutrition. From understanding the role of specific nutrients in renal health to providing practical tips on ingredient substitutions, this cookbook serves as an invaluable companion for those taking their first steps towards a plant-based, kidney-conscious lifestyle.

What sets this cookbook apart is its unwavering commitment to inclusivity. It recognizes that every individual's relationship with their kidneys is unique, and it caters to a spectrum of dietary needs and preferences. Whether you're a seasoned chef or a kitchen novice, the recipes in "Harmony in Greens" are crafted with simplicity and clarity in mind, ensuring that the joy of cooking remains accessible to all.

The journey to kidney-friendly vegetarianism is not just about the destination; it's about savoring each step along the way. The cookbook seamlessly weaves together the science of renal nutrition with the artistry of flavors, making the process enjoyable and educational. Through its pages, you'll discover the delicate balance between creating meals that are kind to your kidneys and indulging your taste buds in a symphony of tastes and textures.

As you flip through the cookbook, you'll encounter a diverse array of recipes that showcase the bounty of plant-based ingredients. From savory soups that warm the soul to vibrant salads that celebrate the colors of nature, each dish is a testament to the idea that nourishing your kidneys doesn't mean compromising on taste. The recipes are meticulously curated to bring out the best in every ingredient, proving that kidney-friendly meals can be both health-conscious and a culinary delight.

"Harmony in Greens" extends an invitation to explore the world of kidney-friendly vegetarianism with curiosity and enthusiasm. It's not just a cookbook; it's a mentor that empowers you to make informed choices about what goes into your body. Through engaging narratives, nutritional insights, and step-by-step guides, it transforms the kitchen into a classroom where you learn to prioritize your health without sacrificing the pleasures of a good meal.

For those who find solace in the act of preparing food, this cookbook becomes a companion in the kitchen, guiding you through the creation of meals that resonate with both your taste buds and your kidneys. It bridges the gap between intention and action, offering practical solutions for incorporating kidney-friendly practices into your daily culinary routine.
In the realm of kidney-friendly vegetarian cookbooks, "Harmony in Greens" stands out as a testament to the idea that taking care of your kidneys can be a flavorful, enjoyable journey. As you embark on this adventure, let the pages of this cookbook be your compass, guiding you towards a harmonious blend of health and gastronomic

satisfaction. Get ready to embark on a culinary exploration that not only nourishes your body but also feeds your soul – a journey where kidney-friendly and vegetarian are seamlessly united in the art of delicious living.

CHAPTER ONE

Understanding Kidney Health

- Importance of Kidneys

The kidneys, two bean-shaped organs located on either side of the spine, play a vital role in maintaining the overall health and well-being of the human body. Their importance extends far beyond merely filtering waste and excess fluids from the blood. The intricate functions performed by the kidneys are integral to various physiological processes, making them essential for life.
One of the primary functions of the kidneys is the filtration of blood to remove waste products and excess fluids. This process ensures the body maintains a proper balance of electrolytes and other essential substances. The waste products, including urea and creatinine, are then excreted as urine. Without this filtration process, toxins would accumulate in the bloodstream, leading to a range of health issues and, ultimately, organ failure.
Beyond waste elimination, the kidneys play a crucial role in regulating blood pressure. They achieve this by adjusting the volume of blood and the concentration of sodium and other electrolytes in the body. The renin-angiotensin-aldosterone system, a complex hormonal cascade involving the

kidneys, helps control blood pressure by influencing blood vessel constriction and fluid balance. Furthermore, the kidneys are central to the maintenance of a stable acid-base balance in the body. They excrete hydrogen ions and reabsorb bicarbonate, ensuring that the blood remains within a narrow pH range. This acid-base equilibrium is vital for the proper functioning of enzymes and other biochemical processes. Imbalances in this system can lead to acidosis or alkalosis, disrupting cellular functions and affecting overall health.

The kidneys also play a pivotal role in the regulation of red blood cell production. They release a hormone called erythropoietin, which causes the bone marrow to start producing red blood cells. Adequate red blood cell levels are crucial for oxygen transport, and any disruption in this process can lead to anemia and a range of associated complications.

Moreover, the kidneys contribute significantly to the metabolism of vitamin D, a key player in calcium homeostasis. Through the conversion of vitamin D into its active form, the kidneys facilitate the absorption of calcium and phosphorus in the intestines. This process is essential for bone health, nerve function, and muscle contraction. A deficiency in vitamin D due to impaired kidney function can result in weakened bones and increased susceptibility to fractures.

The importance of the kidneys becomes particularly evident in cases of kidney disease or failure. Chronic kidney disease (CKD) is a progressive condition that can lead to irreversible damage, impairing the organs' ability to carry out their vital functions. Individuals with advanced CKD may require dialysis or kidney transplantation to sustain life.

In conclusion, the kidneys stand as indispensable organs with multifaceted functions crucial for maintaining homeostasis within the body. From waste elimination and blood pressure regulation to acid-base balance and red blood cell production, their impact on overall health cannot be overstated. Recognizing the importance of kidney health underscores the need for preventive measures, early detection of renal disorders, and the promotion of lifestyle choices that support these vital organs in their intricate tasks.

- ## Common Kidney Conditions

Kidney conditions encompass a wide range of disorders that affect the kidneys, vital organs responsible for filtering waste products and excess fluids from the blood to produce urine. Common kidney conditions can result from various factors, including genetic predisposition, infections, autoimmune disorders, and lifestyle choices. Understanding these conditions is crucial for early detection, management, and prevention.

1. Chronic Kidney Disease (CKD):

Chronic Kidney Disease is a prevalent and progressive condition characterized by the gradual loss of kidney function over time. Diabetes and hypertension are leading causes of CKD, emphasizing the importance of managing these conditions to prevent kidney damage. As CKD advances, complications such as electrolyte imbalances, anemia, and bone disease can arise. Early detection through regular screenings, along with lifestyle modifications and medication management, is crucial in slowing the progression of CKD.

2. Kidney Stones:

Kidney stones are solid deposits that form in the kidneys from mineral and acid salts. These crystals can cause severe pain as they pass through the urinary tract. Dehydration, diet high in certain minerals, and genetic factors contribute to stone

formation. Treatment involves pain management,
increased fluid intake, and, in some cases, medical
procedures to break down or remove larger stones.

3. Urinary Tract Infections (UTIs):

While UTIs can affect any part of the urinary
system, they commonly involve the kidneys.
Bacterial infections can lead to inflammation and
compromise kidney function. Prompt treatment with
antibiotics is crucial to prevent the spread of
infection and potential damage to the kidneys.
Maintaining good hygiene and staying hydrated are
essential in preventing UTIs.

4. Polycystic Kidney Disease (PKD):

PKD is a genetic disorder characterized by the
growth of fluid-filled cysts in the kidneys, leading to
an increase in organ size and potential impairment
of function. This condition often progresses slowly
and may lead to complications such as high blood

pressure and kidney failure. Regular monitoring, blood pressure control, and supportive care are essential components of managing PKD.

5. Glomerulonephritis:

Glomerulonephritis involves inflammation of the glomeruli, the tiny blood vessels in the kidneys responsible for filtering waste and excess fluids. This condition can be acute or chronic and may result from infections, autoimmune diseases, or certain medications. Symptoms may include blood in the urine, swelling, and hypertension. Treatment aims to address the underlying cause and manage symptoms to prevent further kidney damage.

6. Acute Kidney Injury (AKI):

AKI is a sudden and rapid decline in kidney function, often caused by factors like severe infections, dehydration, or exposure to nephrotoxic substances. Timely identification and intervention are crucial to prevent long-term damage. Treatment involves addressing the underlying cause, fluid management, and supportive care.

7. Nephrotic Syndrome:

Nephrotic syndrome is characterized by the presence of protein in the urine, low blood protein levels, high cholesterol, and swelling. Various kidney diseases can lead to nephrotic syndrome, impacting the kidneys' ability to filter blood properly. Treatment may involve medications to control proteinuria, diuretics to manage swelling, and addressing the underlying kidney disease.

In conclusion, understanding common kidney conditions is essential for promoting kidney health and preventing complications. Regular health check-ups, maintaining a healthy lifestyle, and addressing risk factors contribute to the overall well-being of the kidneys. Early detection and appropriate management play a pivotal role in preserving kidney function and preventing the progression of these conditions.

The Role of Diet in Kidney Function:

The role of diet in kidney functions is pivotal, as the kidneys play a crucial role in maintaining overall health by filtering waste products and excess fluids from the blood. A balanced and kidney-friendly diet is essential to support these vital organs and prevent the development or progression of kidney diseases.

Firstly, controlling the intake of sodium is paramount. High sodium levels can lead to increased blood pressure, putting additional strain on the kidneys. A diet rich in processed and packaged foods tends to be high in sodium, so opting for fresh fruits and vegetables, as well as using herbs and spices for flavoring instead of salt, is advisable. This helps in managing blood pressure and reducing the risk of kidney damage.

Fluid intake is another critical aspect. While staying hydrated is essential, excessive fluid consumption can burden the kidneys, especially in individuals with kidney problems. Striking a balance between staying adequately hydrated and not overloading the kidneys is key. Monitoring urine color can serve as a simple indicator; pale yellow urine generally signifies proper hydration.

Protein intake must also be moderated. While protein is vital for the body, excessive consumption can strain the kidneys, particularly in individuals with existing kidney issues. High-quality protein sources like lean meats, poultry, fish, and plant-based proteins such as beans and legumes are preferable. Monitoring protein intake is especially crucial for those with kidney disease, as their ability to eliminate waste products is compromised.

Controlling phosphorus and potassium levels is important for individuals with kidney disease. Foods high in phosphorus, such as dairy products and certain nuts, should be limited. Similarly, potassium-rich foods like bananas, oranges, and tomatoes need to be moderated, as imbalances can disrupt heart rhythm and muscle function, exacerbating kidney problems.

Maintaining a healthy weight is linked to better kidney function. Obesity is a risk factor for kidney disease, and weight management through a balanced diet and regular exercise can contribute to overall kidney health. A diet rich in fruits, vegetables, and whole grains while limiting saturated and trans fats supports weight management and reduces the risk of developing kidney-related complications.

Certain nutrients play a specific role in kidney health. Antioxidants, found in fruits and vegetables, help protect the kidneys from oxidative stress.

Vitamin D is crucial for calcium absorption, and its deficiency can lead to mineral imbalances and bone problems, affecting kidney function. Adequate intake of these nutrients through a well-rounded diet is essential.

Individuals with kidney stones need to be mindful of their diet to prevent stone formation. Increasing fluid intake to dilute substances in the urine that lead to stones and reducing the consumption of oxalate-rich foods, such as beets and chocolate, can be beneficial. Additionally, limiting salt and animal protein intake helps manage specific types of kidney stones.

In conclusion, a well-balanced and kidney-friendly diet is integral to supporting optimal kidney function and preventing kidney-related issues. Monitoring sodium, protein, fluid, phosphorus, and potassium intake, along with maintaining a healthy weight, contributes to overall kidney health. Tailoring dietary choices to individual needs, especially for those with existing kidney conditions, is crucial. By adopting a proactive approach to nutrition, individuals can play an active role in safeguarding their kidney functions and promoting long-term well-being.

CHAPTER TWO

Kidney-Friendly Nutrition Basics

- ○ Essential Nutrients for Kidney Health

1. Water:

Adequate hydration is fundamental for kidney health. Water helps in the efficient elimination of waste products through urine and prevents the formation of kidney stones. Dehydration can lead to concentrated urine, increasing the risk of stone formation and potential kidney damage.

2. Electrolytes:

Maintaining a balance of electrolytes, such as sodium, potassium, and calcium, is essential for kidney function. Sodium regulates fluid balance, while potassium is crucial for nerve and muscle function. Calcium plays a role in blood clotting and bone health. Imbalances in these electrolytes can lead to kidney stones and other complications.

3. Protein:

Protein is a vital nutrient for the body, but excessive protein intake can strain the kidneys. It's essential to strike a balance. High-quality, lean protein sources like fish, poultry, and plant-based proteins provide essential amino acids without overburdening the kidneys.

4. Omega-3 Fatty Acids:

Walnuts, flaxseeds, and fatty fish like salmon are good sources of omega-3 fatty acids, which have anti-inflammatory qualities. Inflammation is linked to kidney disease progression, and incorporating omega-3s into the diet may help mitigate this risk.

5. Antioxidants:

Antioxidants, including vitamins A, C, and E, help combat oxidative stress in the body. Kidneys are vulnerable to oxidative damage due to their high blood flow. Fruits and vegetables, especially those with vibrant colors, are rich sources of antioxidants that can benefit kicney health.

6. Vitamin D:

For the body to absorb calcium, which is necessary for healthy bones, vitamin D is required. Kidneys play a role in activating vitamin D, and its deficiency can contribute to kidney disease. Exposure to sunlight and dietary sources like fatty fish and fortified foods can help maintain adequate vitamin D levels.

7. B Vitamins:

B vitamins, including B6, B12, and folic acid, play a role in red blood cell production and help in maintaining healthy nerve function. Deficiencies in these vitamins can contribute to anemia and kidney problems.B vitamins can be found in lean meats, whole grains, and leafy greens..

8. Magnesium:

Magnesium supports muscle and nerve function, bone health, and blood pressure regulation. It also helps in the elimination of waste and toxins from the body. Magnesium is abundant in whole grains, nuts, seeds, and leafy green vegetables.

9. Phosphorus:

While phosphorus is essential for bone health, too much can be detrimental to individuals with kidney issues. People with kidney disease may need to limit phosphorus intake. Dairy products, nuts, seeds, and whole grains are common sources of phosphorus.

10. Low-Glycemic Carbohydrates:

For the kidneys to remain healthy, blood sugar levels must remain constant. Opting for low-glycemic carbohydrates, such as whole grains, legumes, and vegetables, can help prevent complications associated with diabetes, a leading cause of kidney disease.

In conclusion, a well-balanced and nutrient-rich diet is crucial for maintaining kidney health. Hydration, electrolyte balance, appropriate protein intake, and a variety of vitamins and minerals contribute to overall kidney function. It's essential to tailor dietary choices to individual health needs and consult with healthcare professionals, especially for those with existing kidney conditions. Prioritizing these essential nutrients can go a long way in promoting kidney health and preventing the onset or progression of kidney disease.

- ○ **Reading Food Labels for Kidney Diet**

Reading food labels is crucial for individuals following a kidney-friendly diet, as it empowers them to make informed choices about the foods they consume. For those with kidney issues, understanding the nutritional content of packaged items is essential for managing sodium, potassium, and phosphorus intake.

Kidney health is closely tied to dietary considerations, and food labels provide a wealth of information to help navigate these restrictions. When examining a food label, the first step is to focus on serving size. Often, people overlook this aspect and consume more than the recommended serving, inadvertently increasing their nutrient intake.

Sodium is a primary concern for individuals with kidney problems, as excessive intake can lead to

fluid retention and elevated blood pressure.
Reading the "sodium" section on food labels helps
in monitoring salt intake. It's essential to choose
items labeled as "low sodium" or "sodium-free"
whenever possible. Pay attention to the absolute
sodium content per serving, as this gives a clear
picture of how much sodium is in the food.

Potassium is another mineral that requires close
monitoring in a kidney-friendly diet. While
potassium is essential for various bodily functions,
excessive levels can be harmful for those with
compromised kidney function.Moderate
consumption is advised while consuming foods
high in potassium, such as oranges and
bananas.Reading the potassium content on food
labels aids in avoiding items that may contribute to
elevated potassium levels.

Phosphorus is yet another nutrient that needs
careful consideration. Elevated phosphorus levels
can be detrimental to kidney health, leading to bone

and heart issues. Food labels provide information on phosphorus content, helping individuals with kidney concerns make wise dietary choices. Often, processed and packaged foods contain added phosphorus in the form of preservatives or additives, making it crucial to identify and limit such items.

Understanding the ingredient list is equally important. The main component is mentioned first and the other ingredients are written in descending order of weight. For those with kidney issues, it's beneficial to choose products with simpler ingredient lists, avoiding items with phosphorus additives or high sodium content. Being aware of various names for sodium and phosphorus additives is essential for accurate label interpretation.

Nutrient content claims on food labels can also guide individuals in making kidney-friendly choices. Phrases such as "low sodium," "no added phosphorus," or "kidney-friendly" can be indicators that the product aligns with dietary restrictions. However, it's crucial not to rely solely on these claims; a thorough examination of the entire label ensures a comprehensive understanding of the food's nutritional profile.

The importance of monitoring protein intake is amplified for those with kidney issues. Protein is a vital component of a balanced diet, but excessive protein can strain compromised kidneys. Reading the protein content on food labels helps individuals strike a balance, ensuring they meet their nutritional needs without overburdening their kidneys. Choosing lean protein sources and incorporating plant-based proteins can be beneficial for those on a kidney-friendly diet.

Caloric content is another aspect to consider when reading food labels. Managing weight is often a priority for individuals with kidney concerns, and understanding the energy density of foods aids in achieving this goal. Opting for nutrient-dense, lower-calorie options supports overall health and well-being.

Educating oneself about various label terminology is an integral part of deciphering food labels for a kidney-friendly diet. Terms like "reduced," "low," and "free" have specific definitions regulated by food authorities. For instance, a "low sodium" product typically contains 140 milligrams or less of sodium per serving. Familiarizing oneself with these definitions ensures accurate interpretation and informed decision-making.

In conclusion, reading food labels is a fundamental skill for individuals following a kidney-friendly diet. It empowers them to manage their nutrient intake, particularly regarding sodium, potassium, phosphorus, protein, and calories. By paying attention to serving sizes, ingredient lists, and nutrient content claims, individuals can make wise dietary choices that support kidney health. Taking the time to understand food labels ultimately

contributes to a more informed and proactive

approach to managing kidney-related dietary

restrictions.

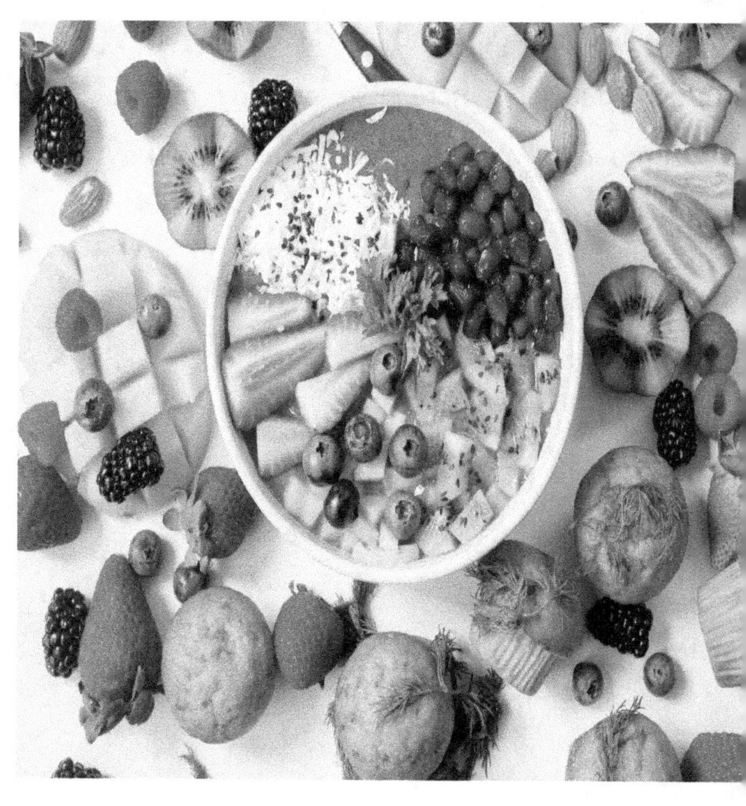

CHAPTER THREE

Getting Started with a Vegetarian Kidney-Friendly Diet

- Transitioning to a Plant-Based Diet:

Transitioning to a plant-based diet can have profound effects on overall health, including benefits for kidney function. As more people recognize the importance of dietary choices in maintaining well-being, the shift towards plant-based eating has gained popularity. In this comprehensive exploration, we will delve into the impact of a plant-based diet on kidney health, addressing key considerations and potential advantages.

Understanding Kidney Health:

The kidneys play a crucial role in filtering waste products and excess fluids from the blood to form urine. For general health, kidney function must be maintained at its best. Diets rich in animal proteins can sometimes lead to the formation of kidney stones and contribute to the progression of kidney disease. Plant-based diets, on the other hand, are often associated with a lower risk of these complications.

Reducing Oxalate Intake:

One noteworthy aspect of transitioning to a plant-based diet is managing oxalate intake. Oxalates are naturally occurring compounds found in many plant foods, and in excess, they can contribute to kidney stone formation. However, it's important to note that not all plant-based foods have high oxalate levels. By diversifying food choices and being mindful of oxalate-rich sources like spinach and beets, individuals can mitigate potential risks.

Balancing Macronutrients:

A well-rounded plant-based diet can provide an excellent balance of macronutrients essential for kidney health. Plant proteins, found in legumes, tofu, and whole grains, offer an alternative to animal proteins without the saturated fats and cholesterol that can stress the kidneys. Additionally, incorporating a variety of colorful fruits and vegetables ensures a rich supply of antioxidants, which may protect against kidney damage.

Managing Phosphorus Levels:

For those with kidney issues, managing phosphorus intake is crucial. While plant-based foods generally contain less absorbable phosphorus than animal-based counterparts, it's still important to be mindful of high-phosphorus plant foods like nuts and seeds. Working with a healthcare professional or nutritionist can help individuals tailor their plant-based diet to meet specific kidney health needs.

Beneficial Nutrients in Plant-Based Foods:

Plant-based diets are inherently rich in nutrients that support kidney health. Potassium, found in fruits, vegetables, and legumes, helps regulate blood pressure and balance fluids in the body. Fiber, abundant in whole grains, fruits, and vegetables, promotes overall digestive health and may assist in managing blood sugar levels, a crucial consideration for individuals with kidney disease.

Hydration and Kidney Function:

Adequate hydration is fundamental for kidney function. Plant-based diets, often comprised of water-rich foods like fruits and vegetables, contribute to overall hydration. Emphasizing water intake alongside a plant-based diet further supports kidney health by aiding in the flushing out of toxins.

Potential Challenges and Considerations:

While transitioning to a plant-based diet can offer numerous benefits for kidney health, it's important to approach this shift thoughtfully. Some individuals may face challenges, such as ensuring sufficient protein intake and addressing potential nutrient deficiencies. Consulting with a healthcare professional or registered dietitian can help tailor a plant-based diet to individual needs, addressing any concerns and ensuring a well-rounded nutritional profile.

Conclusion:

In conclusion, transitioning to a plant-based diet can positively impact kidney health by reducing the risk of kidney stones, supporting overall kidney function, and provicing essential nutrients. However, it's crucial to approach this dietary shift with awareness, considering factors such as oxalate intake, macronutrient balance, and individual health conditions. With proper planning and guidance, embracing a plant-based lifestyle can be a rewarding journey towards improved kidney health and overall well-being.

- ## Assessing Personal Dietary Needs:

Assessing personal dietary needs in relation to kidney health is a critical aspect of maintaining overall well-being. The kidneys play a vital role in filtering and excreting waste products from the blood, regulating fluid balance, and managing electrolyte levels. Therefore, tailoring one's diet to support optimal kidney function is essential for preventing complications and promoting long-term health.

To assess personal dietary needs in the context of kidney health, it's crucial to comprehend the primary functions of the kidneys. These bean-shaped organs filter blood, removing waste products and excess fluids to form urine. They also help regulate blood pressure, electrolyte balance, and the production of red blood cells. When kidneys are compromised, either due to chronic conditions like diabetes or hypertension or acute issues like infections, dietary adjustments become paramount.

Assessing Current Dietary Habits:

Start by evaluating current dietary habits. Keep a food diary to track daily intake, paying attention to the types and amounts of food consumed. This provides a baseline for identifying potential areas of concern and helps healthcare professionals or nutritionists tailor recommendations to individual needs.

Monitoring Sodium Intake:

Sodium plays a significant role in kidney health, as excessive intake can contribute to high blood pressure, leading to kidney damage over time. Assessing personal dietary needs involves monitoring and reducing sodium consumption. This includes limiting processed foods, canned goods, and restaurant meals, as they often contain hidden salt. Opting for fresh, whole foods and using herbs and spices for flavoring can be effective strategies.

Balancing Fluid Intake:

Kidneys regulate fluid balance, and assessing personal dietary needs involves maintaining an appropriate fluid intake. For individuals with compromised kidney function, fluid restrictions may be necessary to prevent fluid buildup in the body. However, those with healthy kidneys should ensure an adequate intake to support overall hydration.

Managing Protein Intake:
Although an excessive protein diet might cause renal strain, protein is necessary for good health overall. Assessing personal dietary needs involves finding the right balance. Individuals with kidney issues may benefit from consulting a healthcare professional to determine an appropriate protein intake that meets their nutritional needs without overburdening the kidneys.

Considering Phosphorus and Potassium Levels:
Phosphorus and potassium are minerals that need attention in kidney health. Elevated levels of these minerals can lead to complications. Assessing personal dietary needs involves identifying foods rich in phosphorus and potassium and moderating their consumption. This often includes limiting dairy, nuts, and certain fruits and vegetables.

Incorporating Kidney-Friendly Foods:
A kidney-friendly diet emphasizes nutrient-dense, whole foods that support overall health. This includes incorporating fruits and vegetables with lower potassium content, such as apples, berries, and cauliflower. Additionally, choosing lean protein sources like poultry, fish, and eggs can help manage protein intake.

Customizing Dietary Plans:
Individuals with kidney issues have unique needs, and assessing personal dietary requirements involves customization. Consulting with a registered

dietitian or healthcare professional specializing in renal nutrition can provide personalized guidance. These experts can create tailored dietary plans considering individual health status, medical history, and lifestyle factors.

Adapting to Dietary Restrictions:

For those with advanced kidney disease, dietary restrictions may become more stringent. Assessing personal dietary needs involves adapting to these restrictions while still maintaining a balanced and enjoyable diet. This may require creative cooking methods, exploring new recipes, and being mindful of ingredient choices.

Regular Monitoring and Adjustments:

Assessing personal dietary needs is an ongoing process. Regular monitoring of kidney function through blood tests and check-ups helps in making necessary adjustments to the diet. Healthcare professionals can analyze these results and modify dietary recommendations accordingly.

Conclusion:

In conclusion, assessing personal dietary needs in the context of kidney health is essential for maintaining overall well-being. Understanding kidney function, monitoring sodium intake, balancing fluid consumption, managing protein intake, considering phosphorus and potassium levels, incorporating kidney-friendly foods, customizing dietary plans, adapting to restrictions, and regularly monitoring and adjusting are key aspects of this assessment. A proactive and individualized approach to nutrition can significantly contribute to the prevention of kidney-related complications and promote a healthier, more fulfilling life.

CHAPTER FOUR

BUILDING BLOCKS OF A BALANCED PLATE

- Plant-Based Protein Sources:

Maintaining kidney health is a vital aspect of overall well-being, and dietary choices play a pivotal role in supporting optimal kidney function. In recent years, the spotlight has increasingly turned toward plant-based diets for their potential benefits, not only for cardiovascular health and weight management but also for kidney wellness. This article delves into the significance of plant-based protein sources in relation to kidney health, exploring various options and their unique contributions.

1. Lower Phosphorus Content

One of the primary considerations for individuals with kidney concerns is the phosphorus content in their diet. High levels of phosphorus can strain the kidneys, particularly when these organs are not functioning at their full capacity. Plant-based proteins, such as those found in legumes (beans, lentils), tofu, and whole grains, generally contain lower phosphorus levels compared to many animal-based proteins. This characteristic makes them valuable choices for those aiming to manage their phosphorus intake and support kidney wellness.

2. Rich in Fiber for Digestive Health

Beyond their protein content, plant-based foods are often rich in dietary fiber—a key component for digestive health. Fiber contributes to regular bowel movements and helps in maintaining stable blood sugar levels. This is especially relevant for individuals with kidney issues, as conditions like diabetes can exacerbate kidney problems. By opting for plant-based protein sources, individuals not only support their kidney health but also address broader concerns related to overall well-being.

3. Legumes: Versatile and Kidney-Friendly

Legumes, including beans, lentils, and chickpeas, emerge as star players in the realm of plant-based proteins with specific benefits for kidney health. These foods are not only low in phosphorus but also boast a favorable nutrient profile, including ample fiber and a variety of essential vitamins and minerals.

Their versatility allows for creative culinary exploration, making it easier for individuals to incorporate kidney-friendly proteins into their daily meals.

4. Nuts and Seeds: Nutrient-Rich Options

Nuts and seeds are nutrient-dense sources of plant-based proteins. While they do contain phosphorus, the form of phosphorus in these foods is bound to fiber. This binding may limit the absorption of phosphorus, potentially easing the burden on the kidneys. Additionally, nuts and seeds provide healthy fats, vitamins, and minerals, contributing to an overall balanced diet that supports not only kidney health but also other aspects of well-being.

5. Tofu and Soy Products: Complete Proteins

Tofu and other soy-based products are integral components of plant-based diets, offering complete proteins containing all nine essential amino acids. For individuals transitioning away from animal products, tofu provides a versatile and protein-rich alternative. However, it's important to note that moderation is key, as excessive protein intake, even from plant sources, may need to be monitored, especially for those with kidney concerns.

6. Quinoa: A Complete Plant-Based Protein

Quinoa stands out among grains as a complete protein source, containing all essential amino acids. This makes quinoa an excellent addition to a plant-based diet, ensuring individuals receive a well-rounded spectrum of amino acids necessary for various bodily functions, including those related to kidney health. Its versatility in the kitchen adds to its appeal, allowing for the creation of diverse and nutritionally balanced meals.

7. Balancing Act and Professional Guidance

While embracing plant-based protein sources can offer numerous benefits for kidney wellness, it's essential to approach dietary changes with a balanced perspective. Variety is key to meeting overall nutritional needs, and individuals should consult healthcare professionals or registered dietitians to tailor their diets to specific requirements. Striking a balance between different plant-based proteins, incorporating a range of vegetables, fruits, and whole grains, ensures a comprehensive nutrient intake that supports kidney health.

In conclusion, plant-based protein sources present a promising avenue for promoting kidney wellness. From legumes and nuts to tofu and quinoa, these options offer not only essential proteins but also a myriad of nutrients that contribute to overall health. However, individualized dietary approaches and professional guidance are crucial to address specific needs and ensure a well-rounded, kidney-friendly diet. By making informed choices and embracing the diverse array of plant-based proteins available, individuals can take proactive steps toward nurturing their kidney health and fostering a holistic sense of well-being.

Choosing low-potassium vegetables is crucial for creating a kidney-friendly vegetarian cookbook that supports renal health. Kidneys play a vital role in maintaining electrolyte balance, and individuals with kidney issues often need to manage their potassium intake. Crafting a cookbook tailored to this need involves thoughtful selection of vegetables that are not only delicious but also kidney-friendly.

To begin with, it's essential to understand why potassium is a concern for those with kidney problems. Potassium is a mineral that helps nerves and muscles communicate, but impaired kidneys may struggle to filter it out efficiently. Elevated potassium levels can lead to serious health complications, including irregular heartbeats. Therefore, a kidney-friendly vegetarian cookbook must focus on vegetables with lower potassium content.

One excellent choice is leafy greens with lower potassium levels. Spinach, kale, and Swiss chard are nutrient-rich options that are lower in potassium compared to alternatives like beet greens or collard greens. Incorporating these greens into salads, stir-fries, or soups can add depth of flavor and nutritional value without excessively raising potassium levels.

Cruciferous vegetables are another category to explore. Broccoli, cauliflower, and cabbage are not only low in potassium but also provide fiber and essential vitamins. These vegetables offer versatility, fitting into various recipes like roasted vegetable medleys, creamy soups, or as a side dish. Their mild flavors make them adaptable to different culinary styles, enhancing the cookbook's overall appeal.

Root vegetables, despite their earthy flavors, can vary in potassium content. Opting for lower potassium options like carrots, turnips, or radishes can maintain the cookbook's kidney-friendly focus. These vegetables can be roasted, steamed, or included in stews to add depth and heartiness to vegetarian dishes. It's important to be mindful of portion sizes to control potassium intake effectively.

Tomatoes, commonly used in many vegetarian dishes, can be included but in moderation. While tomatoes are a good source of vitamins and antioxidants, they also contain potassium. Using them sparingly or opting for tomato products with lower potassium levels, such as tomato sauce rather than fresh tomatoes, can help strike a balance between flavor and renal health.

Bell peppers, both colorful and flavorful, are excellent choices for a kidney-friendly vegetarian cookbook. Red, yellow, and green peppers are lower in potassium compared to some other vegetables, making them versatile additions to salads, fajitas, or stuffed pepper recipes. Their vibrant colors can enhance the visual appeal of dishes, making them more enticing for those following a renal-friendly diet.

Incorporating legumes into the cookbook is a wise choice for both protein and fiber. However, not all legumes have the same potassium content. Lentils, chickpeas, and black beans are lower in potassium compared to options like kidney beans or edamame.

These legumes can be featured in main dishes, soups, or salads, providing a satisfying and kidney-friendly protein source.

When seasoning recipes, herbs and spices become invaluable. Opting for low-potassium herbs like parsley, thyme, or dill can add depth and flavor without compromising renal health. Experimenting with various spice blends allows for the creation of diverse and flavorful dishes, catering to different tastes while keeping potassium levels in check.

In conclusion, crafting a kidney-friendly vegetarian cookbook involves thoughtful consideration of vegetable choices. By selecting low-potassium options and being mindful of portion sizes, one can create delicious and nutritious recipes that support renal health. From leafy greens to cruciferous vegetables, root vegetables, tomatoes in moderation, bell peppers, and kidney-friendly legumes, the possibilities are vast. Pairing these vegetables with kidney-conscious herbs and spices ensures a well-rounded and appealing cookbook that promotes both culinary enjoyment and renal wellness.

- Healthy Fats for Kidney Health

In the context of a kidney-friendly vegetarian cookbook, understanding and incorporating healthy fats is crucial for supporting kidney health. While it's common to associate a low-fat diet with kidney health, it's important to differentiate between unhealthy fats and those that offer essential nutrients. Healthy fats can contribute to overall well-being, and carefully selecting them enhances the nutritional value of vegetarian recipes tailored for individuals with kidney concerns.

Avocado, rich in monounsaturated fats, stands out as a kidney-friendly choice. It adds a creamy texture to dishes without overloading them with saturated or trans fats. Avocado can be incorporated into salads, spreads, or used as a topping for various dishes, providing a satisfying and heart-healthy source of fats.

Olive oil, particularly extra virgin olive oil, is another excellent option. Packed with monounsaturated fats and antioxidants, it not only enhances the flavor of recipes but also offers anti-inflammatory benefits. Using olive oil as a base for salad dressings, sautéing vegetables, or drizzling over roasted dishes introduces healthy fats while maintaining a kidney-conscious approach.

Nuts and seeds, in moderation, provide a nutrient-rich source of healthy fats. Walnuts, flaxseeds, and chia seeds are high in omega-3 fatty acids, which have anti-inflammatory properties. Including these in a kidney-friendly vegetarian cookbook can add a crunchy element to salads, cereals, or desserts, boosting both flavor and nutritional content.

Coconut oil, though high in saturated fat, can be used sparingly for its distinct flavor. While it's not the primary source of fats in a kidney-friendly diet, incorporating small amounts in recipes like curries or desserts can contribute a unique taste without significantly impacting overall fat intake.

Fatty fish alternatives for vegetarians include chia seeds and flaxseeds. These tiny seeds are rich in omega-3 fatty acids, promoting heart and kidney health. Grinding them and adding them to smoothies, oatmeal, or using them as an egg substitute in recipes can offer a plant-based omega-3 boost.

Nut butters, such as almond or peanut butter, can be included in moderation. These spreads provide a creamy texture and a dose of healthy fats. Using them as a base for sauces, dips, or incorporating them into desserts allows for versatility in a kidney-friendly vegetarian cookbook.

Dairy or dairy alternatives can contribute healthy fats. Opting for low-fat or fat-free versions of yogurt, milk, or cheese ensures a protein source without excess saturated fats. These dairy products can be integrated into recipes like smoothies, soups, or casseroles, enhancing both flavor and nutritional value.

Flavorful seeds like pumpkin seeds, also known as pepitas, offer a nutrient-dense addition to kidney-friendly recipes. They can be sprinkled on salads, added to granola, or included in vegetable dishes, providing a crunchy texture along with healthy fats, protein, and minerals.

In summary, incorporating healthy fats into a kidney-friendly vegetarian cookbook involves a thoughtful selection of sources. Avocado, olive oil, nuts, seeds, coconut oil in moderation, and plant-based omega-3 sources like chia seeds and flaxseeds contribute to a diverse and nutritious range of fats. Balancing these fats with other kidney-friendly ingredients ensures that the cookbook not only promotes renal health but also provides delicious and satisfying meal options for individuals with specific dietary needs.

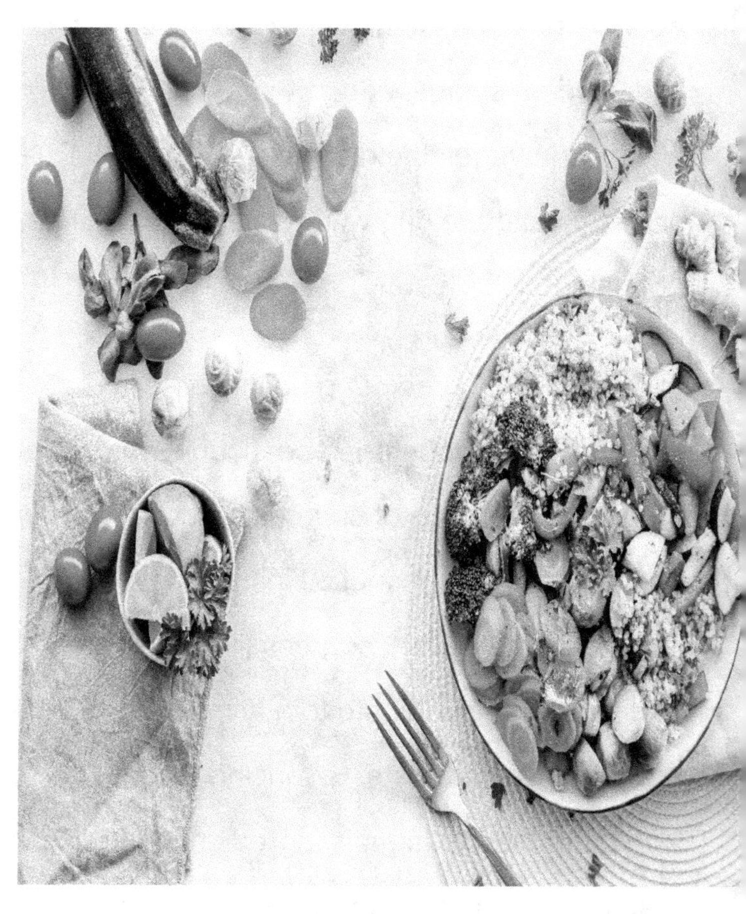

CHAPTER FIVE

DELICIOUS AND NUTRIENT-PACKED BREAKFAST

Overnight Oats with Berries

Creating a kidney-friendly overnight oats recipe with berries involves thoughtful consideration of ingredients that support renal health. Overnight oats are not only convenient but also offer an opportunity to incorporate nutritious elements into the diet. Let's explore a comprehensive recipe that is both delicious and tailored to promote kidney wellness.

Ingredients:

- 1/2 cup old-fashioned oats (low in phosphorus)
- 1/2 cup unsweetened almond milk (low in potassium)
- 1/4 cup fresh blueberries (antioxidant-rich)
- 1/4 cup fresh strawberries, sliced (low in potassium)
- 1 tablespoon chia seeds (omega-3 fatty acids)
- 1 tablespoon chopped almonds (low in potassium, high in healthy fats)
- 1/2 teaspoon cinnamon (adds flavor without sodium)
- 1/2 teaspoon vanilla extract (adds sweetness without added sugars)
- Optional: 1 teaspoon honey or maple syrup (use sparingly for sweetness)

Instructions:

Combine Dry Ingredients:

1. In a mason jar or airtight container, mix
    the old-fashioned oats, chia seeds,
    chopped almonds, and cinnamon.
    These ingredients provide a balance of
    fiber, healthy fats, and essential
    nutrients without overloading on
    phosphorus or potassium.

Add Wet Ingredients:

2. Add vanilla essence and unsweetened
    almond milk. Almond milk is a
    kidney-friendly alternative to dairy, and
    vanilla extract adds natural sweetness
    without resorting to high-sugar options.

Incorporate Berries:

3. Gently fold in the fresh blueberries and
    sliced strawberries. Berries are rich in
    antioxidants, vitamins, and fiber, making
    them excellent choices for kidney health
    without contributing excessive
    potassium.

Stir and Refrigerate:

4. Mix all ingredients thoroughly, ensuring an even distribution of flavors. Seal the container and refrigerate overnight. This enables the flavors to combine and the oats to absorb the liquid.

Serve and Garnish:

5. Stir well the next morning with the oats. If desired, drizzle a small amount of honey or maple syrup for sweetness. However, be mindful of added sugars, and use these sweeteners sparingly.

Top with Extra Berries:

6. Enhance the visual appeal and nutritional content by topping the oats with a few extra fresh berries. This provides a burst of flavor and additional antioxidants.

Enjoy Mindfully:

7. Savour the kidney-friendly overnight oats with berries mindfully, appreciating the combination of textures and flavors. This breakfast option offers a balance of essential nutrients while adhering to the dietary considerations necessary for kidney wellness.

By focusing on low-phosphorus and low-potassium ingredients, incorporating healthy fats from almonds and chia seeds, and leveraging the antioxidant benefits of berries, this comprehensive overnight oats recipe aligns with kidney-friendly principles. It not only provides a delicious breakfast option but also supports overall renal health by avoiding excessive phosphorus and potassium content.

A Vegetable and Feta Omelette can be a kidney-friendly option, considering certain dietary guidelines for kidney wellness. To support kidney health, it's crucial to manage protein, phosphorus, and potassium intake.

- ○ **Vegetable and Feta Omelette**

Ingredients:

1. Eggs: A good source of high-quality protein.
2. Vegetables (such as bell peppers, spinach, and onions): Provide essential vitamins and minerals with lower potassium content.
3. Feta cheese: Moderation is key due to its phosphorus content. Choose a lower phosphorus variety if available.
4. Olive oil: A heart-healthy fat option.

Instructions:

1. Egg Preparation: Use egg whites or a combination of whole eggs and egg whites to reduce phosphorus intake.
2. Vegetables: Choose kidney-friendly vegetables and sauté them in olive oil. Avoid high-potassium vegetables like tomatoes and limit phosphorus-rich ones like mushrooms.
3. Feta Cheese: Use a controlled amount of low-phosphorus feta to add flavor.
4. Cooking Oil: Opt for olive oil for its heart-healthy benefits.

Considerations:

- Portion Control: Keep portions moderate to manage protein intake.
- Salt: Limit salt to help control blood pressure.
- Fluid Intake: Stay adequately hydrated, as it aids kidney function.

Always consult with a healthcare professional or a dietitian for personalized dietary advice based on individual health needs and kidney function.

- Smoothie Bowl Varieties

Smoothie bowls are not only delicious and visually appealing but can also be tailored to support kidney health. When considering kidney wellness, it's crucial to manage nutrient intake, focusing on limited phosphorus and potassium levels. Here, we'll explore a variety of kidney-friendly smoothie bowl options, incorporating ingredients that align with renal dietary guidelines.

1. Berry Bliss Bowl

Ingredients:

- Mixed berries (strawberries, blueberries, raspberries): Low in potassium and high in antioxidants.
- Banana (in moderation): A sweet addition with controlled potassium.

- Greek yogurt (low-phosphorus): Adds creaminess and protein.

- Almond milk (unsweetened): A low-potassium alternative to regular milk.

- Chia seeds (optional): Provide omega-3 fatty acids and fiber.

Instructions:

Blend the berries, banana, Greek yogurt, and almond milk until smooth. Pour into a bowl and top with a sprinkle of chia seeds for added texture.

2. Green Goddess Bowl

Ingredients:

- Spinach or kale: Low-potassium greens rich in vitamins.

- Avocado (in moderation): Adds creaminess with controlled potassium.

- Cucumber: Hydrating and low in potassium.

- Celery: A low-potassium, crunchy addition.

- Parsley or cilantro: Fresh herbs for flavor.

- Coconut water: A potassium-friendly liquid base.

Instructions:

Combine the greens, avocado, cucumber, celery, herbs, and coconut water in a blender. Blend until smooth, pour into a bowl, and garnish with a sprig of fresh herbs.

3. Tropical Delight Bowl

Ingredients:

- Pineapple: Low in potassium and adds natural sweetness.
- Mango (in moderation): A tropical flavor with controlled potassium.
- Coconut milk (unsweetened): A creamy base with moderate potassium.
- Plain or vanilla-flavored protein powder (low-phosphorus): Boosts protein content.
- Shredded coconut (unsweetened): Adds texture.

Instructions:

Blend pineapple, mango, coconut milk, and protein powder until smooth. Pour into a bowl and top with a sprinkle of shredded coconut.

4. Oatmeal Cookie Bowl

Ingredients:

- Cooked and cooled oatmeal (in moderation): A low-phosphorus grain.
- Banana (in moderation): Adds natural sweetness with controlled potassium.
- Almond butter (unsalted): A source of healthy fats and protein.
- Almond milk (unsweetened): A low-potassium liquid base.
- Cinnamon: Adds flavor without additional phosphorus.

Instructions:

Blend oatmeal, banana, almond butter, almond milk, and cinnamon until creamy. Pour into a bowl and garnish with a drizzle of almond butter.

5. Citrus Burst Bowl

Ingredients:

- Oranges or tangerines: Low-potassium citrus fruits.
- Pineapple: Adds sweetness and tropical flair.
- Greek yogurt (low-phosphorus): Adds creaminess and protein.
- Almond milk (unsweetened): A low-potassium alternative to regular milk.
- Flaxseeds (optional): A source of omega-3 fatty acids.

Instructions:

Blend oranges, pineapple, Greek yogurt, almond milk, and flaxseeds until smooth. Pour into a bowl and sprinkle additional flaxseeds on top.

Considerations for Kidney Wellness:

- Portion Control: Keep serving sizes moderate to manage nutrient intake.
- Fluid Intake: Stay hydrated, and consider incorporating hydrating ingredients like water-rich fruits.
- Consult a Dietitian: Individualize your smoothie bowl choices based on specific dietary needs and kidney function.

Incorporating these kidney-friendly smoothie bowls into your diet can add variety while prioritizing renal health. Always consult with a healthcare professional or a registered dietitian for personalized advice tailored to your specific health requirements.

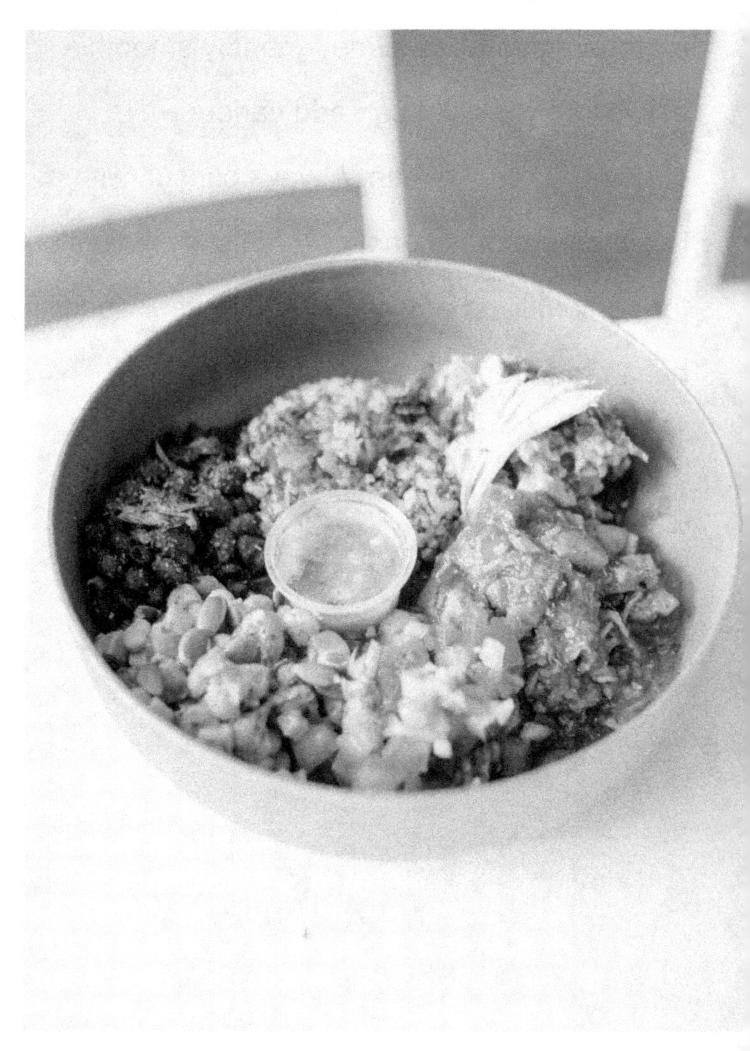

CHAPTER SIX

SATISFYING LUNCH AND DINNER RECIPES

○ Quinoa-Stuffed Bell Peppers

Quinoa-stuffed bell peppers offer a flavorful and nutrient-rich dish that can be tailored to align with kidney wellness guidelines. When focusing on kidney health, it's important to consider nutrient restrictions such as phosphorus and potassium. This dish not only meets these considerations but also provides a wholesome, plant-based source of protein.

Ingredients:

1. Quinoa (rinsed): Quinoa is a high-quality protein source that is lower in

phosphorus compared to many animal-based proteins.

2. Bell Peppers (various colors): Bell peppers are low in potassium, providing a colorful and nutrient-rich base for the dish.
3. Black Beans (canned, drained, and rinsed): A good source of plant-based protein with moderate phosphorus levels.
4. Tomatoes (diced): Tomatoes add a burst of flavor with controlled potassium content.
5. Onion (diced): Onions contribute to flavor without significantly impacting phosphorus or potassium levels.
6. Garlic (minced): Garlic enhances taste while being kidney-friendly.
7. Spinach or Kale (chopped): Leafy greens add vitamins and minerals without elevating phosphorus and potassium levels significantly.
8. Olive Oil: A heart-healthy fat that complements the dish.
9. Spices (cumin, paprika, black pepper): Flavorful additions without contributing to phosphorus or potassium concerns.

10. Low-sodium Vegetable Broth: Enhances the overall taste without adding excessive sodium.

Instructions:

1. Prepare Quinoa:
   - Rinse quinoa thoroughly.
   - Cook quinoa according to package instructions, using low-sodium vegetable broth for added flavor.
2. Prep Bell Peppers:
   - Cut bell peppers in half, removing seeds and membranes.
   - Lightly brush the outer surface with olive oil for a tender texture when baked.
3. Vegetable Saute:
   - In a pan, sauté diced onion and minced garlic in olive oil until translucent.
   - Add chopped spinach or kale, cooking until wilted.
   - Incorporate diced tomatoes and black beans, allowing flavors to meld.

4. Seasoning:
   - Season the vegetable mixture with cumin, paprika, and black pepper to taste.
   - Adjust salt cautiously, considering individual sodium requirements.
5. Combine with Quinoa:
   - Mix the sautéed vegetable mixture with the cooked quinoa, creating a flavorful stuffing.
6. Stuff Bell Peppers:
   - Fill each bell pepper half with the quinoa and vegetable mixture, pressing down gently.
7. Bake:
   - Place stuffed bell peppers in a baking dish.
   - Bake in a preheated oven until peppers are tender.
8. Garnish:
   - For extra taste, garnish with fresh herbs like parsley.

Considerations for Kidney Wellness:

1. Portion Control:

o Enjoy stuffed peppers in moderation to manage protein intake.
   2. Phosphorus Awareness:
        o Quinoa serves as a lower-phosphorus protein option compared to some animal proteins.
   3. Potassium Management:
        o Bell peppers, tomatoes, and spinach provide essential nutrients with controlled potassium levels.
   4. Fluid Intake:
        o Consider hydrating ingredients like tomatoes to support overall fluid balance.
   5. Individual Variations:
        o Adjust ingredients based on individual dietary needs and restrictions.

Conclusion:

Quinoa-stuffed bell peppers offer a wholesome, kidney-friendly meal that combines protein, fiber, and essential nutrients. The dish caters to those mindful of phosphorus and potassium intake, making it suitable for individuals with kidney health considerations. The versatility of this recipe allows for creative variations while adhering to renal dietary guidelines. Always consult with a healthcare professional or a registered dietitian to tailor the recipe to specific health needs and ensure it aligns with individual dietary restrictions. Incorporating such nutrient-dense and kidney-friendly recipes contributes to a balanced and enjoyable approach to maintaining kidney wellness.

- Lentil and Kale Salad

Lentil and Kale Salad can be a nutritious and kidney-friendly choice with the right ingredients. Here's a kidney-conscious recipe along with instructions:

Ingredients:

- One cup cooked and cooled lentils, either green or brown
- 4 cups chopped kale greens with the stems removed
- 1 cup cherry tomatoes, halved
- 1 cucumber, diced
- 1/4 cup red onion, finely chopped
- 1/4 cup fresh parsley, chopped
- 1/4 cup feta cheese, crumbled (optional)
- 2 tablespoons extra-virgin olive oil
- 2 tablespoons balsamic vinegar
- 1 teaspoon Dijon mustard
- Salt and pepper to taste

Instructions:

1. Prepare Lentils:

- Cook lentils according to package instructions. Once cooked, let them cool to room temperature.

2. Massage Kale:

   - In a large mixing bowl, place the chopped kale.
   - Give the kale a little drizzle of olive oil and give it a few minutes of massage.This helps to soften the kale and reduce bitterness.

3. Assemble the Salad:

   - Add the cooled lentils, cherry tomatoes, cucumber, red onion, and fresh parsley to the bowl with kale.

4. Prepare the Dressing:Olive oil, balsamic vinegar, Dijon mustard, salt, and pepper should all be combined in a small bowl.Adjust the seasoning to your taste.

5. Dress the Salad:

   - Over the salad, drizzle with the dressing and mix to fully incorporate.

6. Optional: Add Feta Cheese:

   - For extra taste, top the salad with crumbled feta cheese, if preferred.Be mindful of portion sizes to manage phosphorus intake.

7. Chill Before Serving:Before serving, let the salad cool in the fridge for at least half an hour.This enhances the flavors.

8. Serve and Enjoy:

   - Serve the Lentil and Kale Salad as a refreshing and kidney-friendly side dish or a light meal.

9. Customization:

- Tailor the recipe to your dietary needs by adjusting the quantities or choosing low-phosphorus ingredients.

Notes:

- Phosphorus Awareness:
    - Monitor phosphorus intake by choosing low-phosphorus options, especially if you have kidney concerns.
- Fluid Intake:
    - Enjoy this salad with a glass of water to contribute to your daily fluid intake.
- Consult with a Professional:
    - If you have specific dietary restrictions or concerns related to kidney health, it's advisable to

consult with a healthcare professional or a registered dietitian for personalized guidance.

This kidney-friendly Lentil and Kale Salad not only brings a burst of flavors but also provides a nutrient-rich option that aligns with renal health considerations.

- Eggplant Parmesan

Eggplant Parmesan can be a delicious and kidney-friendly option with a few mindful adjustments. Here's a kidney-conscious recipe along with instructions:

Ingredients:

- 1 large eggplant, sliced into 1/2-inch rounds
- 2 eggs, beaten
- 1 cup whole wheat breadcrumbs
- 1/2 cup grated Parmesan cheese (low-sodium)
- 1 teaspoon dried oregano
- 1 teaspoon dried basil
- 1/2 teaspoon garlic powder
- Salt and pepper to taste
- Olive oil cooking spray
- 2 cups marinara sauce (low-sodium)
- 1 1/2 cups shredded mozzarella cheese (low-sodium)
- Fresh basil for garnish (optional)

Instructions:

Preheat the Oven:

1. Preheat your oven to 375°F (190°C).

2. Prepare the Eggplant:

   - Sprinkle salt on the eggplant slices and let them sit for about 15 minutes. This helps draw out excess moisture.

   - Pat the eggplant slices dry with a paper towel to remove the salt and moisture.

3. Breading the Eggplant:

   - In a bowl, mix breadcrumbs, grated Parmesan, oregano, basil, garlic powder, salt, and pepper.

   - Dip each eggplant slice into the beaten eggs, ensuring both sides are coated.

   - Dredge the eggplant in the breadcrumb mixture, pressing gently to adhere the coating.

4. Bake the Eggplant:

   - Arrange the breaded eggplant slices onto a parchment paper-lined baking sheet.
   - Lightly spray the slices with olive oil cooking spray.
   - Bake in the preheated oven for about 20-25 minutes or until the eggplant is golden brown and tender.

5. Layering the Eggplant Parmesan:

   - Apply a thin layer of marinara sauce to a baking dish.
   - Place a layer of baked eggplant slices on top.
   - Sprinkle mozzarella cheese over the eggplant.

- Repeat the layers until all the ingredients are used, finishing with a layer of mozzarella on top.

6. Bake Until Bubbly:

   - Bake the assembled Eggplant Parmesan in the oven for an additional 20-25 minutes or until the cheese is melted and bubbly.

7. Garnish and Serve:

   - Give the eggplant parmesan a few minutes to settle before slicing.
   - Garnish with fresh basil if desired.

8. Portion Control:

   - Pay attention to portion sizes, as excessive protein and sodium intake can be a concern for kidney health.

9. Customization:

   - Tailor the recipe to your dietary needs by choosing low-sodium or salt-free ingredients.

Notes:

- Sodium Considerations:
  - Opt for low-sodium or salt-free versions of ingredients like breadcrumbs, marinara sauce, and Parmesan cheese to manage sodium intake.
- Fluid Intake:
  - Enjoy this dish with a side of vegetables or a fresh salad to contribute to your daily fluid intake.
- Consult with a Professional:

- If you have specific dietary restrictions or concerns related to kidney health, it's advisable to consult with a healthcare professional or a registered dietitian for personalized guidance.

This kidney-friendly Eggplant Parmesan allows you to savor a classic dish while being mindful of your renal health.

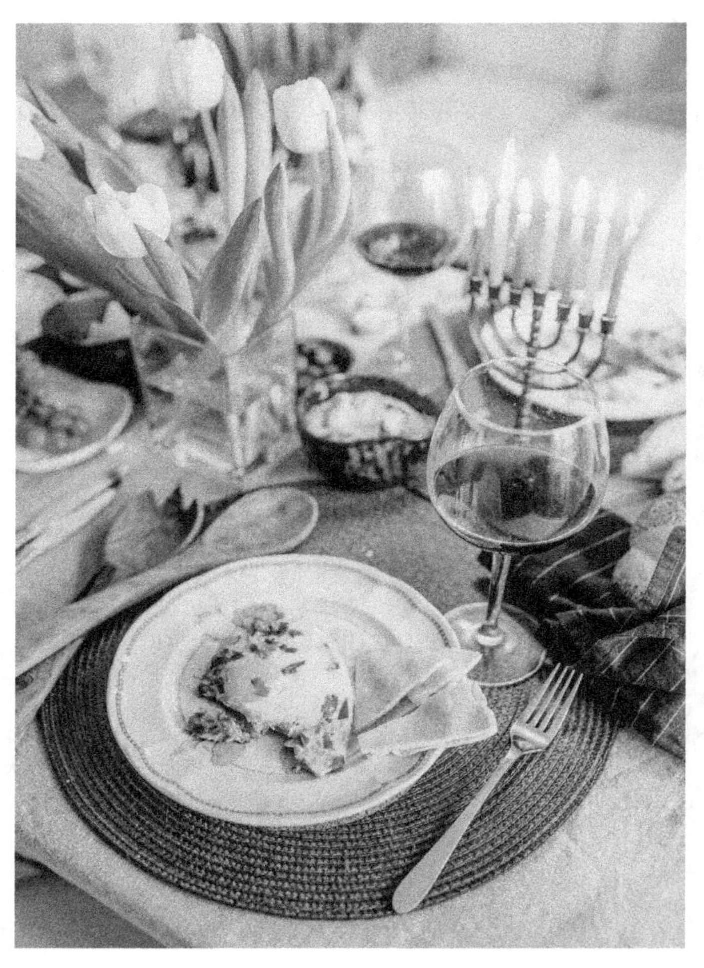

CHAPTER SEVEN

SNACKS AND APPETIZERS

- Roasted Chickpeas

incorporating kidney-friendly foods into your diet can play a pivotal role in supporting these vital organs. One such nutritious and delicious option is roasted chickpeas. Packed with protein, fiber, and an array of essential nutrients, chickpeas can be transformed into a crunchy snack that aligns with kidney-friendly dietary guidelines.

Nutritional Benefits of Chickpeas for Kidney Health:

Chickpeas, also known as garbanzo beans, are a nutrient-dense legume that provides a healthy dose of plant-based protein. This is essential for individuals with kidney concerns, as it helps meet protein needs without burdening the kidneys with excessive waste products. Additionally, chickpeas are rich in fiber, promoting digestive health and aiding in the management of blood sugar levels—both crucial aspects for those with kidney issues.

Roasted Chickpeas Recipe:

Ingredients:

- Two cans of washed and drained chickpeas, 15 ounces each
- 2 tablespoons olive oil
- 1 teaspoon salt
- 1 teaspoon garlic powder
- 1 teaspoon onion powder
- 1 teaspoon cumin
- 1/2 teaspoon paprika

Instructions:

1. Preheat the Oven: Preheat your oven to 400°F (200°C).
2. Dry Chickpeas: Pat the drained chickpeas dry with a paper towel. Removing excess moisture is crucial for achieving a crispy texture.
3. Seasoning: In a bowl, combine the chickpeas with olive oil, salt, garlic powder, onion powder, cumin, and paprika. Toss until the chickpeas are evenly coated with the seasoning.
4. Spread on Baking Sheet: Spread the seasoned chickpeas in a single layer on a baking sheet. Ensure they are not overcrowded to allow even roasting.
5. Roast in the Oven: Place the baking sheet in the preheated oven and roast for 25-30 minutes or until the chickpeas are golden brown and crunchy. Shake the pan halfway through the cooking time to promote even roasting.
6. Cool Before Serving: Allow the roasted chickpeas to cool before serving. They will continue to crisp up as they cool down.

Kidney-Friendly Considerations:

1. Moderate Protein Content: Chickpeas offer a moderate protein content, suitable for those following a kidney-friendly diet. However, individual protein needs may vary, so it's advisable to consult with a healthcare professional or a registered dietitian.
2. Low in Sodium: By controlling the amount of salt in the seasoning, you can manage the sodium content, crucial for individuals with kidney issues. Opting for herbs and spices to enhance flavor can be a healthier alternative.
3. Hydration is Key: As with any kidney-friendly diet, staying adequately hydrated is essential. The fiber content in chickpeas requires sufficient water intake for optimal digestion.

In conclusion, roasted chickpeas present a delightful and kidney-friendly snack option. Rich in protein, fiber, and an array of essential nutrients, this recipe allows individuals to enjoy a tasty treat while supporting their kidney health.For individualized nutritional guidance based on unique health needs, always seek the counsel of a certified dietitian or other healthcare provider.

- Guacamole with Veggie
  Sticks

Guacamole with Veggie Sticks is a delightful and kidney-friendly snack that not only satisfies your taste buds but also provides essential nutrients for maintaining kidney health. This recipe focuses on incorporating ingredients that are low in potassium and phosphorus, making it suitable for individuals with kidney concerns.

Guacamole Recipe for Kidney Health

Ingredients:

- 3 ripe avocados
- 1 small red onion, finely diced
- 2 medium tomatoes, diced
- 1 clove garlic, minced
- 1 lime, juiced
- 1 tablespoon cilantro, chopped
- Salt and pepper to taste

Veggie Sticks:

- Carrot sticks
- Celery sticks
- Cucumber slices
- Bell pepper strips

Instructions:

1. Avocado Selection:

Start by choosing ripe avocados. A ripe

avocado should give slightly when applied

gently.

2. Prepare Vegetables:

Wash and chop the tomatoes, red onion, garlic,

and cilantro. Set them aside in separate bowls.

3. Avocado Preparation:

Scoop the flesh from the avocados into a

mixing bowl after cutting them in half and

removing the pit.

4. Mash Avocados:

To get the desired consistency, mash the avocados with a fork. Some people enjoy a chunkier guacamole, while others prefer it smoother.

5. Add Lime Juice:

Squeeze the juice of one lime into the mashed avocados. Lime not only adds a zesty flavor but also helps prevent the avocados from browning.

6. Incorporate Vegetables:

Gently fold in the diced tomatoes, finely diced red onion, minced garlic, and chopped cilantro into the mashed avocados.

7. Season to Taste:

Add salt and pepper to taste. Remember that kidney-friendly recipes often require moderation in salt, so start with a little and adjust according to your preference.

8. Veggie Sticks Preparation:
Wash and cut carrot sticks, celery sticks, cucumber slices, and bell pepper strips. These crunchy veggies add a refreshing element to the dish.

9. Serve and Enjoy:
Arrange the guacamole in a bowl, surrounded by the colorful assortment of veggie sticks. The vibrant presentation enhances the overall appeal of the dish.

Kidney Health Considerations:

1. Limit Potassium:

Avocados are a good source of potassium, but this recipe keeps the portion size moderate. It's essential to be mindful of potassium intake for individuals with kidney issues.

2. Phosphorus Management:
Tomatoes contain some phosphorus, but their incorporation in this recipe is balanced. Individuals on a low-phosphorus diet should monitor their overall phosphorus intake.

3. Hydration:
Lime juice not only enhances flavor but also contributes to hydration, which is crucial for kidney health.

4. Customization:
This recipe is adaptable to individual dietary restrictions. Consult with a healthcare professional or a dietitian to personalize it based on specific kidney health needs.

In conclusion, Guacamole with Veggie Sticks is

a kidney-friendly snack that combines flavors

and textures while being mindful of nutrient

restrictions. Enjoy this delicious and nutritious

treat as part of a balanced diet that supports

overall kidney health.

Hummus:

Hummus is a versatile and kidney-friendly dip made primarily from chickpeas, which are a good source of plant-based protein. To make a kidney-friendly hummus, consider the following recipe:

Ingredients:

- 1 can (15 ounces) of low-sodium chickpeas, drained and rinsed
- 2 tablespoons tahini (sesame seed paste)
- 2 tablespoons olive oil
- 1 clove garlic, minced
- 2 tablespoons fresh lemon juice
- 1/2 teaspoon cumin
- Salt and pepper to taste

Instructions:

1. In a food processor, combine chickpeas, tahini, olive oil, garlic, lemon juice, and cumin.
2. Add water as required to blend until smooth and reach the desired consistency.
3. Season with salt and pepper to taste.

This hummus recipe focuses on using low-sodium chickpeas and includes minimal added salt. Adjusting salt intake is essential for kidney health, as excessive sodium can contribute to high blood pressure and fluid retention.

Whole Grain Crackers:

Pairing hummus with whole grain crackers enhances the snack's nutritional profile by adding fiber and complex carbohydrates. Here's a kidney-friendly whole grain cracker recipe:

Ingredients:

- 1 cup whole wheat flour
- 1/2 cup oats
- 1/4 cup flaxseeds
- 1/4 cup sesame seeds
- 1/4 cup olive oil
- 1/2 cup water
- 1/2 teaspoon salt

Instructions:

1. Preheat the oven to 350°F (175°C).
2. In a food processor, combine whole wheat flour, oats, flaxseeds, sesame seeds, olive oil, water, and salt.
3. Pulse until the mixture forms a dough.

4. Roll out the dough on a floured surface and cut into desired cracker shapes.
5. Place the crackers on a baking sheet and bake for 15-20 minutes or until golden brown.

Using whole wheat flour and oats in this cracker recipe provides fiber without an excess of phosphorus, which is an important consideration for those with kidney issues.

When enjoying hummus and whole grain crackers for kidney health, it's crucial to be mindful of portion sizes to avoid overloading on nutrients that may be restricted. Additionally, consulting with a healthcare professional or a registered dietitian can provide personalized advice based on individual kidney health needs.

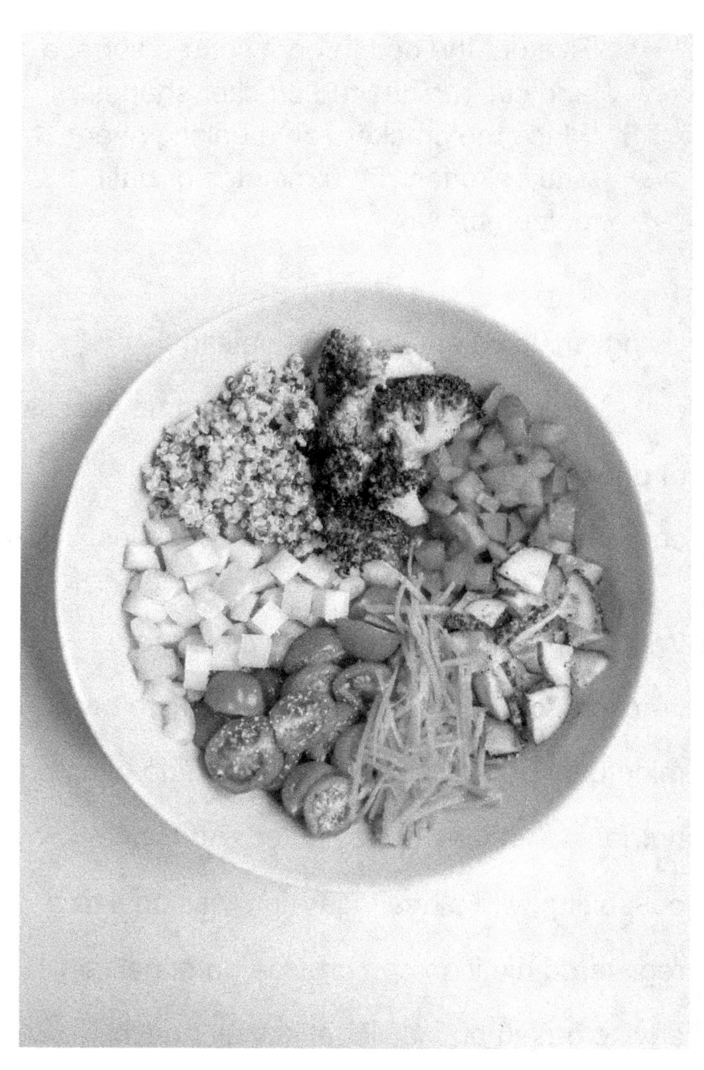

CHAPTER EIGHT

HYDRATION AND KIDNEY-FRIENDLY BEVERAGES

- Importance of Water

Water is a fundamental element for sustaining life, and its importance extends to the intricate mechanisms of kidney wellness. The kidneys, two bean-shaped organs situated on either side of the spine, play a pivotal role in maintaining the body's internal equilibrium. Water, being a universal solvent, is integral to the proper functioning of these vital organs.

One of the primary functions of the kidneys is to filter waste products and toxins from the bloodstream, forming urine as a means of excretion. Adequate water intake is crucial for this filtration process. When the body is well-hydrated, the blood volume remains stable, allowing the kidneys to effectively remove waste and maintain a proper balance of electrolytes. This optimal blood volume ensures that the kidneys can perform their filtration duties without unnecessary strain.

Furthermore, water plays a key role in preventing the formation of kidney stones. Kidney stones are crystallized deposits that can develop when the urine becomes too concentrated, leading to the precipitation of minerals. Insufficient water intake contributes to the concentration of urine, making it more conducive to stone formation. By drinking an ample amount of water, individuals dilute their urine, reducing the risk of mineral crystallization and the subsequent development of kidney stones. This preventive aspect underscores the importance of water in preserving kidney health.

Proper hydration is also essential for preventing urinary tract infections (UTIs), which can adversely affect kidney function. The urinary tract, including the bladder and urethra, is susceptible to bacterial infections. Water helps flush out bacteria from the urinary system, reducing the likelihood of infection. Inadequate water intake can lead to stagnant urine, providing an environment conducive to bacterial growth. A well-hydrated body, on the other hand, promotes the continual flushing of bacteria, minimizing the risk of UTIs and safeguarding the kidneys from potential harm.

Beyond its role in specific kidney-related conditions, water contributes to overall metabolic processes that indirectly impact renal wellness. Hydration supports digestion, nutrient absorption, and the transportation of essential substances throughout the body. The kidneys rely on these systemic processes to receive nutrients and oxygen for their own well-being. Thus, maintaining an adequate water balance ensures that the kidneys receive the necessary resources to function optimally.

In addition to preventing kidney stones and urinary tract infections, water aids in the regulation of blood pressure. The kidneys play a pivotal role in blood pressure regulation by adjusting the volume of blood and the concentration of electrolytes. When the body is adequately hydrated, blood volume remains stable, allowing the kidneys to maintain optimal blood pressure. Proper blood pressure is crucial for preserving the structural integrity of the kidneys and preventing long-term damage associated with hypertension.

In conclusion, the importance of water in relation to kidney wellness cannot be overstated. From facilitating the filtration of waste products to preventing the formation of kidney stones and urinary tract infections, water is a cornerstone of renal health. Its impact extends beyond the kidneys, influencing overall bodily functions that are intricately connected to renal well-being. As we recognize the vital role water plays in sustaining life, we concurrently acknowledge its indispensable role in maintaining the health and functionality of one of the body's most vital organs—the kidneys.

- Herbal Tea Blends

1. Dandelion Detox Blend:
    - Ingredients:
        - 1 tablespoon dried dandelion leaves
        - 1 teaspoon nettle leaves
        - 1 teaspoon marshmallow root
    - Instructions:
        - For five to seven minutes, steep the herbs in boiling water.
        - Strain and enjoy. Dandelion promotes kidney function, while nettle and marshmallow root offer anti-inflammatory benefits.

2. Cranberry Cleanse Tea:
    - Ingredients:
        - 1 tablespoon dried cranberries
        - 1 teaspoon parsley leaves
        - 1 teaspoon hibiscus petals
    - Instructions:
        - Boil the ingredients in water for 10 minutes.

- Strain and drink. Cranberries are known for preventing urinary tract infections, and parsley supports kidney health.

3. Ginger Lemon Flush:
    - Ingredients:
        - 1 tablespoon fresh ginger slices
        - 1 tablespoon dried lemon peel
        - 1 teaspoon turmeric powder
    - Instructions:
        - Simmer the ingredients for 15 minutes.
        - Strain and sip. Ginger aids digestion, lemon supports detoxification, and turmeric has anti-inflammatory properties.

4. Minty Kidney Soother:
    - Ingredients:
        - 1 tablespoon dried mint leaves
        - 1 teaspoon coriander seeds
        - 1 teaspoon fennel seeds
    - Instructions:

- Steep the herbs in hot water for 8 minutes.
- Strain and enjoy. Mint has a cooling effect, while coriander and fennel help flush out toxins.

5. Green Tea Basil Boost:
   - Ingredients:
     - 1 green tea bag
     - 1 tablespoon fresh basil leaves
     - 1 teaspoon chamomile flowers
   - Instructions:
     - Brew the green tea and add basil and chamomile.
     - Let it steep for 3-5 minutes. Green tea is rich in antioxidants, basil supports kidney function, and chamomile has calming properties.

These herbal tea blends not only provide hydration but also incorporate herbs known for their kidney-supporting properties. Remember to consult with a healthcare professional before introducing new herbs into your routine, especially if you have existing health conditions.

○ Infused Water Ideas

Infused water can be a refreshing and healthful way to support kidney wellness. Staying hydrated is crucial for kidney function, and adding natural flavors to your water can make it more enjoyable. Here are some infused water ideas along with recipes and instructions to promote kidney health.

1. Cucumber Mint Splash:
    - Ingredients: 1 cucumber (sliced), a handful of fresh mint leaves, 1 lemon (sliced).

o Instructions: Combine cucumber, mint, and lemon slices in a pitcher. Fill with water and let it infuse in the refrigerator for at least 2 hours. This blend is not only hydrating but also contains antioxidants from mint and hydration benefits from cucumber.

2. Berry Citrus Burst:
   o Ingredients: 1 cup mixed berries (strawberries, blueberries, raspberries), 1 orange (sliced).
   o Instructions: In a pitcher, add the mixed berries and orange slices. Fill with water and refrigerate for a few hours. Berries provide a dose of vitamins and antioxidants, while citrus adds a refreshing twist.

3. Lemon Ginger Detox:
   o Ingredients: 1 lemon (sliced), 1-inch ginger (sliced).
   o Instructions: Combine lemon and ginger slices in a pitcher, fill with water, and let it infuse overnight. Lemon provides a citric kick and vitamin C, while ginger adds anti-inflammatory properties, promoting kidney health.

4. Watermelon Basil Bliss:
   o Ingredients: 2 cups watermelon chunks, a handful of fresh basil leaves.

- Instructions: Mix watermelon chunks and basil leaves in a pitcher, fill with water, and let it chill for a few hours. Watermelon is hydrating, and basil brings a unique flavor along with potential anti-inflammatory benefits.

5. Pineapple Mint Delight:
   - Ingredients: 1 cup pineapple chunks, a handful of fresh mint leaves.
   - Instructions: Combine pineapple chunks and mint leaves in a pitcher, fill with water, and refrigerate. Pineapple provides a tropical sweetness, and mint adds a refreshing element while potentially supporting digestion.

6. Herbal Infusion:
   - Ingredients: 1 sprig of rosemary, 1 sprig of thyme, 1 lemon (sliced).
   - Instructions: Place rosemary, thyme, and lemon slices in a pitcher, fill with water, and let it infuse for a few hours. Herbs like rosemary and thyme can contribute to antioxidant and anti-inflammatory effects.

7. Apple Cinnamon Spice:
   - Ingredients: 1 apple (sliced), 1 cinnamon stick.
   - Instructions: Combine apple slices and a cinnamon stick in a pitcher, fill with water, and refrigerate. Apples provide hydration, and cinnamon

adds a hint of spice along with potential anti-inflammatory properties.

8. Cherry Lime Zest:
    - Ingredients: 1 cup cherries (pitted), 2 limes (sliced).
    - Instructions: Mix cherries and lime slices in a pitcher, fill with water, and let it infuse for a few hours. Cherries bring natural sweetness, and lime adds a zesty flavor along with vitamin C.

Incorporating these infused water ideas into your daily routine not only helps in staying hydrated but also adds essential vitamins, minerals, and antioxidants that can support kidney health. Experiment with different combinations to find your favorite flavors while nourishing your body. Remember to stay consistent and make water a fundamental part of your kidney wellness journey. Cheers to your health!

CHAPTER NINE

MEAL PLANNING AND PREPARATION

- Weekly Meal Plans

Day 1:

Breakfast: Quinoa Breakfast Bowl

- Cooked quinoa with almond milk, topped with sliced strawberries, a handful of blueberries, and a sprinkle of chia seeds.

Lunch: Lentil and Vegetable Stew

- Ingredients: Lentils, carrots, bell peppers, spinach, vegetable broth, cumin, garlic, onion.
- Instructions: Sauté garlic and onion, add lentils, vegetables, and broth. Simmer until lentils are tender.

Dinner: Baked Sweet Potato and Broccoli

- Ingredients: Sweet potatoes, broccoli, olive oil, salt, pepper.
- Instructions: Bake sweet potatoes until tender, steam broccoli, and top with a drizzle of olive oil.

Day 2:

Breakfast: Green Smoothie Bowl

- Ingredients: Spinach, banana, mixed berries, almond milk.
- Instructions: Blend ingredients until smooth. Almond slices and pumpkin seeds should be placed on top.

Lunch: Chickpea Salad

- Ingredients: Chickpeas, cucumber, cherry tomatoes, feta cheese, lemon vinaigrette.
- Instructions: Mix ingredients in a bowl and toss with lemon vinaigrette.

Dinner: Eggplant Stir-Fry

- Ingredients: Eggplant, tofu, bell peppers, snap peas, soy sauce.
- Instructions: Stir-fry ingredients in a pan, season with soy sauce, and serve over brown rice.

Day 3:

Breakfast: Greek Yogurt Parfait

- Ingredients: Greek yogurt, granola, peaches, flaxseeds.
- Instructions: Layer ingredients in a glass or bowl.

Lunch: Spinach and Mushroom Quiche

- Ingredients: Whole-grain crust, spinach, mushrooms, low-fat cheese, eggs.
- Instructions: Bake a quiche with the mentioned ingredients.

Dinner: Cauliflower and Lentil Curry

- Ingredients: Cauliflower, lentils, curry spices, coconut milk.
- Instructions: Cook lentils, simmer with cauliflower, curry spices, and coconut milk.

Day 4:

Breakfast: Mixed Berry Oatmeal

- Ingredients: Steel-cut oats, mixed berries, yogurt, honey.
- Instructions: Cook oats, top with berries, yogurt, and a drizzle of honey.

Lunch: Avocado and Black Bean Wrap

- Ingredients: Whole-grain wrap, avocado, black beans, lettuce, salsa.

- Instructions: Assemble ingredients in a wrap.

Dinner: Zucchini Noodles with Pesto

- Ingredients: Zucchini noodles, basil pesto, cherry tomatoes.
- Instructions: Toss zucchini noodles with pesto, add cherry tomatoes.

Day 5:

Breakfast: Chia Seed Pudding

- Ingredients: Chia seeds, almond milk, kiwi, shredded coconut.
- Instructions: Mix chia seeds with almond milk, refrigerate, and top with kiwi and coconut.

Lunch: Quinoa and Vegetable Buddha Bowl

- Ingredients: Quinoa, roasted vegetables, hummus, tahini dressing.
- Instructions: Assemble a bowl with the mentioned ingredients.

Dinner: Stuffed Bell Peppers

- Ingredients: Bell peppers, quinoa, black beans, corn, tomatoes.
- Instructions: Stuff peppers with a mix of cooked quinoa, black beans, corn, and tomatoes.

Day 6:

Breakfast: Banana Walnut Muffins

- Ingredients: Whole-grain muffin mix, ripe bananas, chopped walnuts.
- Instructions: Bake muffins according to the package, adding bananas and walnuts.

Lunch: Spinach and Lentil Soup

- Ingredients: Lentils, spinach, tomatoes, vegetable broth, garlic, onion.
- Instructions: Cook lentils with vegetables and broth until tender.

Dinner: Grilled Portobello Mushrooms

- Ingredients: Portobello mushrooms,
  marinade (olive oil, garlic, herbs).
- Instructions: Marinate mushrooms, grill,
  and serve with roasted sweet potatoes.

Day 7:

Breakfast: Fruit Salad with Cottage Cheese

- Ingredients: Mixed fruit salad, low-fat
  cottage cheese.
- Instructions: Combine fruits, serve with
  a side of cottage cheese.

Lunch: Brown Rice and Vegetable Stir-Fry

- Ingredients: Brown rice, kidney-friendly
  vegetables, tofu, soy sauce.
- Instructions: Stir-fry ingredients, season
  with soy sauce, and serve over brown
  rice.

Dinner: Asparagus and Lemon Risotto

- Ingredients: Arborio rice, asparagus,
  lemon zest, Parmesan cheese.

- Instructions: Cook risotto with asparagus, lemon zest, and Parmesan cheese.

Remember to customize portions based on your dietary needs, and consult with a healthcare professional or dietitian to ensure this meal plan aligns with your kidney health requirements. Enjoy your delicious and kidney-friendly vegetarian meals!

- ○ Batch Cooking Tips

Batch cooking can be a game-changer for individuals prioritizing kidney wellness. By planning and preparing meals in advance, you not only save time but also ensure that your dietary choices align with maintaining kidney health. Here are some distinctive batch cooking tips tailored specifically for kidney wellness.

Mindful Ingredient Selection:

1. When embarking on batch cooking for kidney wellness, prioritize ingredients that are kidney-friendly. Opt for low-phosphorus options such as lean proteins like chicken or turkey, and incorporate a variety of colorful vegetables to maximize nutrient intake.

Phosphorus Management:

2. Kidney health often involves monitoring phosphorus intake. Choose fresh, whole foods over processed ones, as they generally contain lower levels of phosphorus. Additionally, consider using phosphate-free cooking methods, such as boiling, to further reduce phosphorus content.

Fluid Balance:

3. Maintaining proper fluid balance is crucial for kidney function. Prepare soups and stews with limited salt content to help regulate fluid levels. Use herbs and spices to enhance flavor without relying on excessive salt, promoting a kidney-friendly and delicious batch-cooked meal.

Portion Control:

4. Batch cooking facilitates portion control, a key aspect of managing kidney health. Divide meals into appropriate serving sizes to avoid overconsumption of nutrients that may strain the kidneys. This practice not only supports kidney wellness but also simplifies meal planning.

Diverse Protein Sources:

5. Incorporate a variety of protein sources into your batch-cooked meals. Beans, lentils, and tofu can be excellent alternatives to animal proteins, providing essential nutrients without overloading the kidneys with excessive protein content. To guarantee a balanced diet, switch up your protein sources.

Low-Potassium Choices:

6. For individuals with kidney concerns, monitoring potassium intake is essential. Choose low-potassium fruits and vegetables, such as apples, berries, and cauliflower, to maintain a kidney-friendly balance. Batch cooking allows you to strategize and incorporate these choices into your meals systematically.

Pre-soaking Techniques:

7. If incorporating beans or legumes, consider pre-soaking them before batch cooking. This simple step can help reduce the potassium and phosphorus content, making these ingredients more kidney-friendly while enhancing their digestibility.

Frozen Produce Convenience:

8. Leverage the convenience of frozen fruits and vegetables in your batch cooking endeavors. Frozen options retain their nutritional value and can be more budget-friendly, ensuring you always have kidney-friendly ingredients readily available.

Labeling and Rotation:

9. Properly label your batch-cooked meals with preparation dates to track freshness and avoid consuming items past their prime. Implement a rotation system in your freezer to ensure that older meals are used first, maintaining the nutritional quality of your kidney-conscious creations.

Consultation with a Dietitian:

10. Individual dietary needs can vary significantly. Before embarking on a batch cooking journey for kidney wellness, consult with a registered dietitian or healthcare professional. They can provide personalized advice, taking into account specific health conditions and nutritional requirements.

Incorporating these batch cooking tips into your routine not only simplifies meal preparation but also contributes to kidney wellness. By being mindful of ingredient choices, portion sizes, and cooking methods, you can enjoy delicious and nourishing meals that support overall kidney health.

- Freezing Kidney-Friendly Meals

Freezing kidney-friendly meals can be a practical and convenient way to ensure a steady supply of nourishing options for individuals with kidney issues. Managing a renal diet often involves careful consideration of nutrient intake, and freezing meals allows for efficient meal planning while maintaining nutritional value.

1. Benefits of Freezing Kidney-Friendly Meals:

Freezing kidney-friendly meals offers several advantages. Firstly, it promotes time efficiency. Preparing and freezing meals in advance ensures that individuals with kidney concerns have access to quick and wholesome options, reducing the need for frequent cooking. This is particularly valuable for those facing time constraints due to work, family, or health-related reasons.

Secondly, freezing helps in portion control. Renal diets often involve strict monitoring of nutrient intake, including sodium, potassium, and phosphorus. By freezing meals in appropriate portions, individuals can manage their serving sizes more effectively, preventing unintentional overconsumption of restricted nutrients.

2. Suitable Ingredients for Kidney-Friendly Freezer Meals:

Choosing the right ingredients is crucial when preparing freezer-friendly meals for those with kidney concerns. Lean proteins such as chicken, turkey, and fish are excellent choices, as they provide essential amino acids without adding excessive phosphorus. Incorporating a variety of vegetables is essential for vitamins and minerals, while carefully selecting low-potassium options like broccoli, cauliflower, and bell peppers.

Whole grains like quinoa and brown rice can contribute to the fiber content of meals, aiding in digestive health. Additionally, using herbs and spices for flavor instead of salt is essential in maintaining a low-sodium diet, which is often recommended for kidney health.

3. Meal Ideas for Freezing:

a. Chicken and Vegetable Casserole:

- Ingredients: Lean chicken, low-potassium vegetables, brown rice.
- Season with herbs and spices for flavor.
- Portion into freezer-friendly containers.

b. Salmon Quinoa Bowls:

- Ingredients: Grilled salmon, quinoa, and a mix of kidney-friendly vegetables.
- Drizzle with a low-sodium dressing before freezing.

c. Turkey and Sweet Potato Chili:

- Ingredients: Ground turkey, kidney beans (in limited quantity), sweet potatoes.
- Use kidney-friendly spices for seasoning.
- Divide into portions and freeze for easy reheating.

4. Freezing Techniques:

Proper freezing techniques are essential to maintain the quality of kidney-friendly meals. Allow the prepared dishes to cool completely before freezing to prevent condensation, which can lead to freezer burn. Consider using airtight containers or freezer bags to minimize exposure to air and prevent ice crystals from forming.

Label each container with the date of preparation and reheating instructions to ensure freshness and avoid confusion.

Additionally, investing in a vacuum sealer can help prolong the shelf life of frozen meals by removing excess air.

5. Reheating Instructions:

When reheating frozen kidney-friendly meals, it's crucial to preserve their nutritional value. Use a microwave or oven, and avoid excessive heat to prevent nutrient degradation. Stirring during the reheating process helps distribute heat evenly.

Monitor the sodium, potassium, and phosphorus content of any additional condiments or sauces used during reheating. Opt for low-sodium options to maintain the integrity of the renal diet.

In conclusion, freezing kidney-friendly meals is a practical strategy for individuals managing kidney-related dietary restrictions. By carefully selecting suitable ingredients, employing proper freezing techniques, and following reheating guidelines, individuals can maintain a diverse and nutritious diet while effectively managing their renal health.

CHAPTER TEN

DINING OUT STRATEGIES

- Navigating Restaurant Menus

Navigating restaurant menus with a focus on kidney wellness involves making informed choices to manage potassium, phosphorus, sodium, and fluid intake. Maintaining a kidney-friendly diet is crucial for those with kidney conditions, and when dining out, a thoughtful approach can contribute to better overall health.

Understanding Dietary Restrictions:

People with kidney issues often need to monitor their potassium and phosphorus intake. Elevated levels of these minerals can strain the kidneys. Additionally, limiting sodium is vital to manage blood pressure, which is commonly associated with kidney problems. When navigating a restaurant menu, it's essential to be aware of these dietary restrictions.

Prioritizing Low-Potassium Options:

Potassium is found in various foods, and limiting its intake is crucial for kidney health. While many fruits and vegetables are high in potassium, there are still plenty of low-potassium options available. Opt for salads with lettuce, cucumbers, and green beans. Choose berries, apples, or grapes for dessert, as these fruits are lower in potassium compared to bananas or oranges.

Managing Phosphorus Intake:

Phosphorus is another mineral that individuals with kidney issues need to monitor. It's commonly present in dairy products, nuts, and certain grains. When perusing the menu, consider opting for vegetarian dishes that exclude high-phosphorus ingredients. Choose whole grains like quinoa over rice, and inquire about the preparation methods to ensure lower phosphorus content.

Minding Sodium Levels:

Excessive sodium can contribute to high blood pressure, putting extra strain on the kidneys. When selecting dishes, choose options with minimal added salt. Avoid processed or cured foods, and inquire if the chef can prepare the meal with reduced sodium. Fresh herbs and spices can add flavor without compromising kidney health.

Opting for Kidney-Friendly Proteins:

For those following a vegetarian diet, protein sources become crucial. Legumes, tofu, and plant-based proteins can be excellent choices. However, it's essential to be mindful of portion sizes and preparation methods. Grilled or baked options are preferable to fried alternatives, as they reduce unnecessary fat intake.

Choosing Smart Beverages:

Fluid intake is a key consideration for kidney wellness. While water is the best choice, other beverages can contribute to daily fluid needs. Avoid sugary sodas and opt for herbal teas or infused water for added flavor without added sugars. Be cautious with alcohol, as it can lead to dehydration.

Customizing Your Order:

Tell the server about any dietary limitations without holding back.Many restaurants are willing to accommodate special requests or make adjustments to dishes. Ask for sauces and dressings on the side, so you can control the amount added. Being proactive about your needs ensures a more tailored dining experience.

Sample Kidney-Friendly Menu

Choices:

1. Appetizer:
   - Grilled vegetable skewers
   - Fresh green salad with a low-potassium vinaigrette
2. Main Course:
   - Quinoa-stuffed bell peppers
   - Lentil curry with brown rice
3. Dessert:
   - Berry sorbet or a fruit platter

Conclusion

Navigating restaurant menus with kidney wellness in mind involves strategic choices that prioritize low-potassium, low-phosphorus, and low-sodium options. By understanding your dietary restrictions and communicating them to restaurant staff, you can enjoy a satisfying and kidney-friendly dining experience. Making informed decisions about what goes on your plate contributes to the overall well-being of your kidneys and supports a healthier lifestyle.

- Communicating Dietary Needs

Maintaining kidney wellness is crucial for overall health, and dietary choices play a pivotal role in supporting kidney function. Communicating dietary needs in the context of kidney wellness involves understanding the specific dietary restrictions and recommendations that can help manage conditions such as chronic kidney disease (CKD). Individuals with kidney issues must work closely with healthcare professionals, including dietitians and nephrologists, to develop a personalized dietary plan tailored to their needs.

Firstly, it's essential to grasp the significance of dietary adjustments in promoting kidney health. The kidneys play a vital role in filtering waste and excess fluids from the blood, and when they are compromised, certain dietary modifications become imperative. Patients with CKD, for instance, may need to monitor their protein intake, as excessive protein can strain the kidneys. Communicating this aspect involves educating individuals on choosing high-quality protein sources, such as lean meats, poultry, fish, and plant-based options like legumes.

Sodium, another critical element, requires meticulous attention. High sodium levels can contribute to fluid retention and elevated blood pressure, both detrimental to kidney function. Communicating the need to limit sodium intake involves educating individuals about hidden sources of sodium in processed foods and encouraging the use of herbs and spices for flavoring instead. Emphasizing the importance of reading food labels becomes crucial for making informed choices.

Fluid management is equally vital in kidney wellness. Individuals may need to adjust their fluid intake based on their specific kidney condition. Communicating this involves conveying the importance of staying hydrated while being mindful of excessive fluid intake, which can strain the kidneys. Encouraging the use of thirst as a guide for fluid consumption can be an effective way to communicate this aspect of kidney-friendly nutrition.

Phosphorus and potassium are minerals that also demand attention in kidney wellness. High levels of these minerals can disrupt the balance in the body and pose challenges for individuals with compromised kidney function. Communicating the need to monitor phosphorus involves educating individuals about its presence in various foods, especially processed and fast foods. Similarly, guiding individuals on managing potassium intake includes highlighting low-potassium food choices and the importance of portion control.

In communicating dietary needs for kidney wellness, collaboration with healthcare professionals is paramount. Dietitians play a crucial role in translating medical recommendations into practical dietary advice. Communicating with a dietitian allows individuals to receive personalized guidance based on their specific health status, preferences, and cultural considerations. Dietitians can help create meal plans that align with dietary restrictions, ensuring optimal nutrition while safeguarding kidney health.

Moreover, incorporating a multidisciplinary approach involving nephrologists further enhances communication about dietary needs. Nephrologists can provide insights into the progression of kidney disease and collaborate with dietitians to fine-tune dietary recommendations accordingly. This collaborative effort reinforces the importance of a holistic approach to kidney wellness.

Family and community support are integral aspects of effective communication regarding dietary needs for kidney wellness. Educating family members and close friends about the dietary restrictions and preferences of individuals with kidney issues fosters a supportive environment. This involves dispelling misconceptions and promoting awareness to ensure that social gatherings and shared meals align with kidney-friendly choices.

In conclusion, communicating dietary needs in relation to kidney wellness requires a comprehensive understanding of the intricacies involved in managing conditions like CKD. From protein intake to sodium restriction and fluid management, conveying these aspects involves education, collaboration with healthcare professionals, and fostering a supportive community. By integrating these elements, individuals can navigate their dietary journey with a focus on kidney health, contributing to an overall enhanced quality of life.

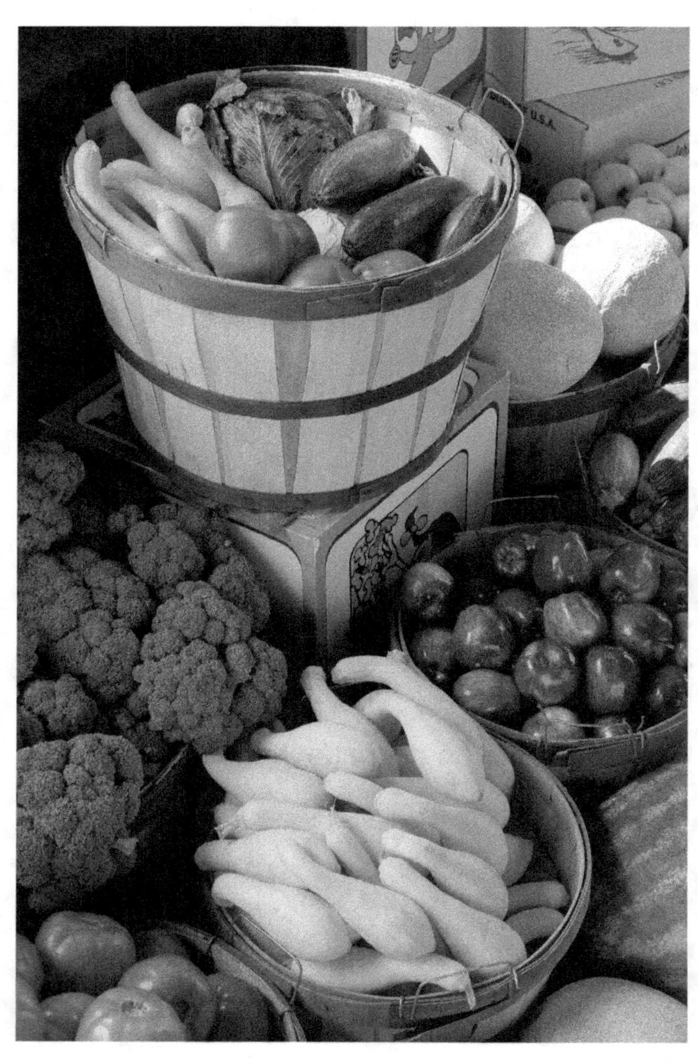

CHAPTER ELEVEN

MANAGING SODIUM AND PHOSPHORUS

- ○ Tips for Reducing Sodium Intake

Reducing sodium intake is a crucial aspect of promoting kidney wellness, especially for individuals managing conditions like chronic kidney disease (CKD). High sodium levels can contribute to fluid retention and elevated blood pressure, both of which can adversely affect kidney function. Implementing practical tips to lower sodium intake involves making informed food choices and adopting mindful eating habits.

1. Read Food Labels: Understanding the sodium content of packaged foods is essential for effective sodium reduction.

Encourage individuals to carefully read food labels to identify high-sodium items. Paying attention to serving sizes is equally important, as some packages may contain multiple servings.

2. Choose Fresh, Whole Foods: Whole foods, such as fruits, vegetables, and unprocessed meats, are naturally lower in sodium. Encourage individuals to focus on incorporating fresh, whole foods into their diet. This not only reduces sodium intake but also provides essential nutrients that support overall health.

3. Limit Processed and Packaged Foods: Processed and packaged foods are often laden with sodium for preservation and flavor enhancement. Advising individuals to limit their consumption of items like canned soups, frozen meals, and processed snacks can significantly contribute to lowering sodium intake.

4. Opt for Low-Sodium Alternatives: Many food products offer low-sodium or sodium-free alternatives. From broths and sauces to canned vegetables, individuals can choose products specifically labeled as low-sodium to reduce their overall sodium intake without sacrificing flavor.

5. Cook at Home: Home-cooked meals provide individuals with greater control over the ingredients and cooking methods. Encourage them to experiment with herbs,

spices, and other flavor enhancers to reduce reliance on high-sodium condiments and seasonings.

6. Rinse Canned Foods: Canned vegetables, beans, and other legumes often come with excess sodium. Advising individuals to rinse these items thoroughly under running water before consumption can help reduce their sodium content significantly.

7. Watch Your Condiments: Certain condiments, such as salad dressings, ketchup, and soy sauce, can contain shockingly high amounts of salt. Suggesting low-sodium or homemade alternatives allows individuals to enjoy flavor without compromising their kidney health.

8. Monitor Restaurant Choices: Dining out can be challenging for those aiming to reduce sodium intake. Recommending that individuals inquire about the sodium content of dishes when eating at restaurants can guide them toward healthier choices. Additionally, opting for grilled or steamed options instead of fried items can contribute to lower sodium consumption.

9. Gradual Reduction: Suddenly eliminating all sources of sodium from the diet may be challenging. Advising individuals to gradually reduce sodium intake allows for a more sustainable and realistic adjustment. This approach can help them adapt to new flavors and develop long-term habits.

10. Keep Yourself Hydrated: Adequate hydration is crucial for kidney health. Drinking an adequate amount of water helps flush excess sodium from the body. Encourage individuals to choose water as their primary beverage and limit the intake of high-sodium drinks like sodas.
11. Educate on Hidden Sodium Sources: Many foods that may not taste particularly salty can still contain significant amounts of sodium. Educate individuals about hidden sodium sources, such as baking soda, baking powder, and some over-the-counter medications. This awareness can contribute to more informed choices.
12. Consult with a Dietitian: Every individual's dietary needs are unique, especially in the context of kidney wellness. Recommending consultation with a registered dietitian allows for personalized guidance based on specific health conditions, lifestyle, and preferences.

In conclusion, reducing sodium intake is a fundamental component of maintaining kidney wellness. By empowering individuals with practical tips such as reading food labels, choosing fresh foods, and being mindful of condiments, they can make informed decisions that align with their dietary goals. Encouraging gradual changes and emphasizing the importance of overall lifestyle adjustments fosters a sustainable approach to sodium reduction, contributing to improved kidney health and overall well-being.

- ○ Phosphorus-Conscious Cooking

Phosphorus-conscious cooking is a critical consideration for maintaining kidney wellness, particularly for individuals facing kidney-related challenges. Phosphorus, a mineral essential for various bodily functions, can become problematic when kidneys struggle to effectively regulate its levels. Understanding which foods contain phosphorus and adopting a mindful approach to meal preparation are crucial components of a kidney-friendly diet.

Several foods are known to be high in phosphorus and should be limited in a phosphorus-conscious cooking regimen. Dairy products, such as milk, cheese, and yogurt, are notable sources of phosphorus. While these are valuable sources of calcium, individuals with kidney concerns must moderate their intake to avoid an excess of phosphorus. Nuts and seeds are another category to be mindful of, as they contain significant amounts of phosphorus. Almonds, sunflower seeds, and pumpkin seeds, while nutritious, should be consumed in moderation.

Animal proteins are often rich in phosphorus, with red meat and organ meats being notable examples. Beef, pork, liver, and kidney meats can contribute substantially to phosphorus intake. Phosphorus-conscious cooking involves choosing leaner cuts of meat and incorporating more plant-based protein sources like legumes, tofu, and tempeh, which generally have lower phosphorus content.

Certain grains and cereals also contain notable levels of phosphorus. Whole grains, bran, and whole wheat products can contribute to phosphorus intake. Phosphorus-conscious cooking encourages opting for refined grains or limiting the consumption of phosphorus-rich grains. Reading labels is essential, as processed foods, including baked goods and cereals, may contain added phosphorus compounds.

Seafood, such as shellfish and fish roe, can be high in phosphorus. While fish is generally a healthy protein source, individuals with kidney concerns should choose varieties lower in phosphorus, such as salmon or trout. Canned fish, particularly those with added sauces or seasonings, may also contribute to higher phosphorus levels.

In addition to recognizing high-phosphorus foods, phosphorus-conscious cooking involves understanding the importance of portion control. Even foods considered moderate in phosphorus can become problematic when consumed in excessive amounts. Managing portion sizes helps individuals strike a balance between obtaining necessary nutrients and avoiding an overload of phosphorus that the kidneys may struggle to process.

Cooking methods play a role in phosphorus-conscious meal preparation. Boiling vegetables and grains can help reduce their phosphorus content, as some phosphorus compounds leach into the cooking water. Rinsing canned beans and vegetables is another practical step to lower phosphorus levels. Incorporating a variety of cooking techniques, such as baking, grilling, and steaming, allows for diverse and flavorful meals without compromising kidney health.

For those actively pursuing phosphorus-conscious cooking, consulting with a registered dietitian is invaluable. A dietitian can provide personalized guidance based on individual health status, preferences, and dietary restrictions. They can assist in creating well-balanced and kidney-friendly meal plans that meet nutritional needs while respecting phosphorus limitations.

In summary, phosphorus-conscious cooking is a key aspect of kidney wellness. Being aware of high-phosphorus foods, practicing portion control, employing suitable cooking methods, and seeking professional guidance are essential components of a kidney-friendly diet. By making informed choices in the kitchen, individuals with kidney concerns can proactively manage their phosphorus intake, supporting overall kidney health and promoting a higher quality of life.

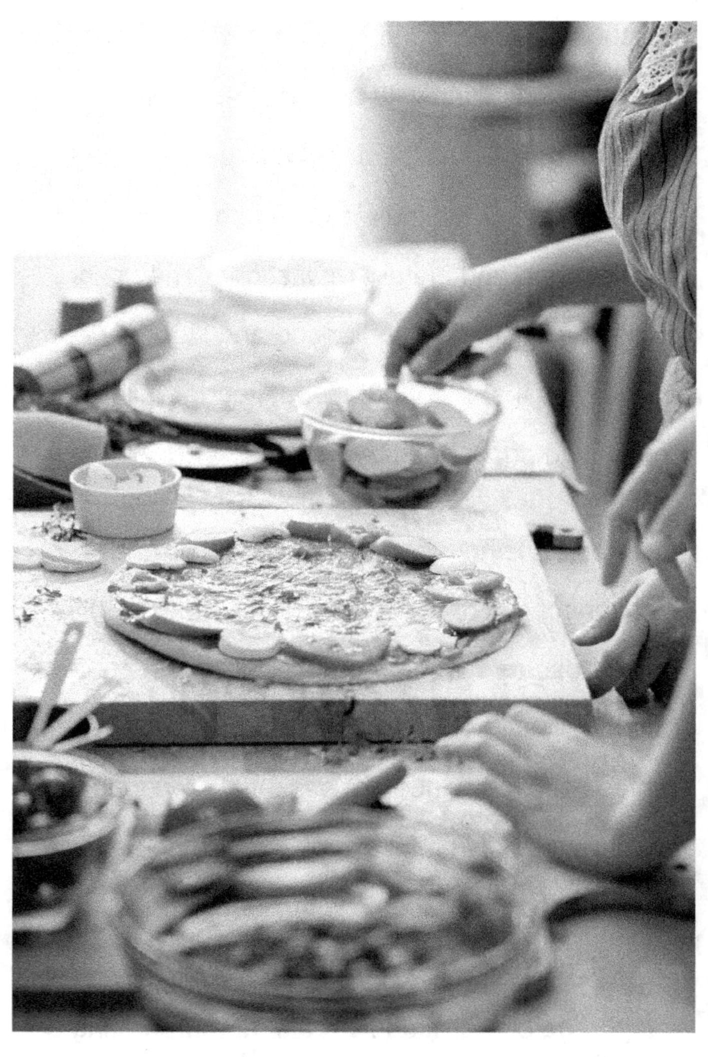

CHAPTER TWELVE

ADDRESSING COMMON CONCERNS

- ○ Vegetarian Protein Myths

Vegetarianism has gained popularity for its perceived health benefits, environmental considerations, and ethical reasons. However, when it comes to kidney wellness, there are several myths surrounding vegetarian protein sources that need clarification. Understanding these myths is crucial for individuals, as misinformation may lead to dietary choices that could impact kidney health.

One common myth is that plant-based proteins lack completeness, meaning they do not provide all essential amino acids necessary for the body. While it is true that some plant-based proteins may be deficient in one or more amino acids, a well-balanced vegetarian diet can easily overcome this limitation. Combining various plant-based protein sources, such as legumes, grains, nuts, and seeds, ensures a diverse amino acid profile, providing the body with the essential building blocks it needs.

Another misconception is that plant-based proteins are insufficient in quantity, making it challenging to meet daily protein requirements. In reality, many plant-based foods are rich in protein, and with proper planning, individuals can easily achieve their protein needs through a vegetarian diet. Lentils, chickpeas, tofu, quinoa, and edamame are just a few examples of protein-packed plant foods that can contribute significantly to daily protein intake.

A prevailing myth suggests that plant-based proteins are harder to digest compared to animal proteins. While it is true that some individuals may experience gas or bloating initially when incorporating more plant-based foods, these symptoms often subside as the digestive system adjusts. Additionally, proper cooking methods, such as soaking, sprouting, or fermenting, can enhance the digestibility of plant-based proteins.

There is a misconception that vegetarian diets lead to nutrient deficiencies, particularly in essential minerals like iron and calcium. In the context of kidney wellness, it's important to note that excessive consumption of animal proteins can burden the kidneys and potentially lead to kidney issues. Plant-based diets, when properly planned, can provide ample nutrients, including iron and calcium, without the negative impact on kidney health associated with high animal protein intake.

Some individuals believe that vegetarian diets lack protein variety, leading to monotony and potential nutritional deficiencies. However, the plant kingdom offers a wide array of protein sources, each with its unique set of nutrients and flavors. From the vast selection of legumes, grains, nuts, seeds, and plant-based protein products, individuals can create diverse and satisfying meals that cater to their protein needs.

Concerns about inadequate protein quality in plant-based diets often stem from misconceptions about protein digestibility and absorption. While plant-based proteins may have slightly lower bioavailability than animal proteins, this doesn't mean they are inadequate. Including a variety of protein sources and complementing them with other nutrient-dense foods enhances overall protein utilization and absorption.

It's a common myth that vegetarian diets lack complete proteins, often leading to the misconception that combining specific plant foods in one meal is necessary. While complementary protein pairing was once thought to be essential in every meal, current nutritional science recognizes that the body efficiently utilizes amino acids over the course of the day. As long as individuals consume a varied diet that includes different plant-based protein sources, they can easily obtain all essential amino acids.

In conclusion, debunking these vegetarian protein myths is crucial for understanding the compatibility of plant-based diets with kidney wellness. A well-planned vegetarian diet can provide abundant, high-quality protein while promoting overall health and reducing the risk of kidney-related issues associated with excessive animal protein intake. By embracing the diversity of plant-based protein sources and dispelling these misconceptions, individuals can confidently pursue a vegetarian lifestyle that supports both their nutritional needs and kidney wellness.

- Handling Cravings and Restrictions.

Handling cravings and dietary restrictions is a significant aspect of maintaining kidney wellness. Individuals with kidney concerns often face unique challenges in managing their diet to support kidney health while addressing cravings for certain foods. Successfully navigating these cravings and restrictions requires a thoughtful and informed approach that focuses on balance, variety, and moderation.

Cravings, whether for salty snacks, sugary treats, or high-phosphorus foods, can pose challenges for individuals with kidney issues. Understanding the reasons behind these cravings is crucial. Sometimes, cravings may be linked to nutritional deficiencies or habits developed over time. For instance, cravings for salty foods might be associated with sodium imbalances, while sweet cravings may indicate a desire for quick energy or emotional satisfaction.

One effective strategy for handling cravings in the context of kidney wellness is to identify and address the root causes. Consulting with a healthcare professional or a registered dietitian can help pinpoint nutritional deficiencies or imbalances, allowing for targeted dietary adjustments. Additionally, adopting healthier alternatives that align with kidney-friendly guidelines can help satisfy cravings without compromising renal health.

An essential aspect of managing cravings and restrictions in kidney wellness is adopting a well-planned and diverse diet. Restricting certain foods doesn't mean sacrificing flavor or variety. Instead, individuals can explore a wide range of kidney-friendly foods and cooking methods to create satisfying meals. Embracing different flavors, textures, and cuisines can make the dietary journey more enjoyable and sustainable.

When it comes to specific dietary restrictions, such as limiting sodium, potassium, or phosphorus intake, careful meal planning becomes crucial. For example, for those watching their sodium levels, reducing processed and packaged foods, using herbs and spices for flavor, and choosing fresh produce can be effective strategies. Similarly, individuals managing phosphorus restrictions might opt for cooking methods that reduce phosphorus content, such as leaching or boiling vegetables.

Education plays a vital role in handling cravings and restrictions for kidney wellness. Understanding the nutritional composition of foods and their impact on kidney function empowers individuals to make informed choices. Reading food labels, being aware of hidden additives, and staying informed about nutrient content contribute to a proactive and knowledgeable approach to dietary management.

It's important to acknowledge that occasional indulgences are a normal part of life, and this holds true for individuals with kidney concerns. Allowing for controlled and mindful treats can help satisfy cravings without jeopardizing kidney health. For example, a small serving of a low-phosphorus dessert or a homemade snack can be integrated into a kidney-friendly diet, providing a sense of balance and enjoyment.

Social support is another valuable resource for individuals managing cravings and restrictions related to kidney wellness. Sharing dietary preferences and restrictions with friends and family helps create a supportive environment. Explaining the importance of adhering to kidney-friendly guidelines can foster understanding and encourage loved ones to make thoughtful choices when planning meals or events.

Meal preparation and cooking at home offer greater control over ingredients and allow for creative adaptations of favorite recipes. Experimenting with herbs, spices, and alternative ingredients can transform familiar dishes into kidney-friendly delights. Engaging in the cooking process enhances the connection with food, making it a positive and enjoyable experience.

In cases where cravings persist or become challenging to manage, seeking guidance from a mental health professional may be beneficial. Emotional and psychological factors often play a role in cravings, and addressing these aspects can contribute to a more holistic approach to kidney wellness. Stress management techniques, mindfulness practices, or counseling can be valuable tools in navigating the emotional aspects of dietary restrictions.

Ultimately, handling cravings and restrictions in relation to kidney wellness is a multifaceted process that involves education, planning, creativity, and support. By focusing on nutrient-rich, kidney-friendly foods, identifying the root causes of cravings, and incorporating occasional treats in a controlled manner, individuals can strike a balance that promotes both renal health and overall well-being. Adopting a positive and proactive mindset, coupled with informed decision-making, empowers individuals to navigate the complexities

of cravings and dietary restrictions while prioritizing

kidney wellness.

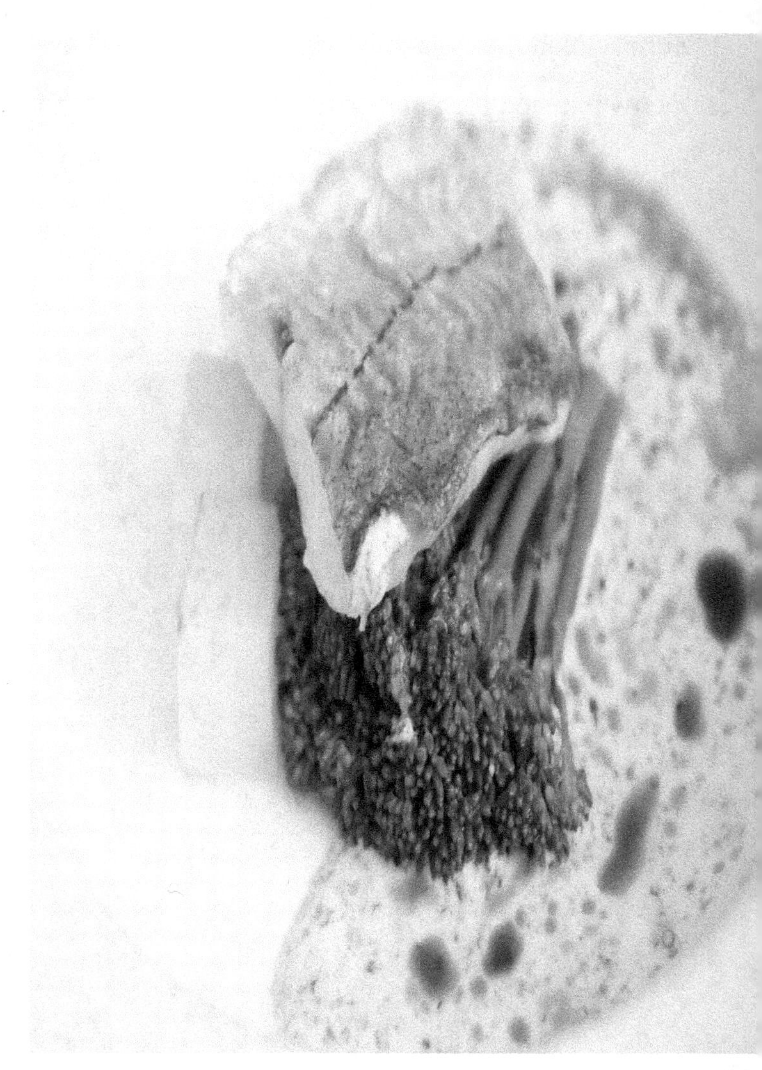

CHAPTER THIRTEEN

EXPERT ADVICES AND Q&A

○ Insights from Nutritionists

Nutritionists play a crucial role in guiding individuals toward a kidney-friendly vegetarian diet, offering valuable insights that promote renal health while adhering to plant-based principles. As more people embrace vegetarianism for various reasons, including ethical, environmental, and health considerations, understanding how to maintain kidney wellness within this dietary framework becomes essential. Here are comprehensive insights from nutritionists on crafting a kidney-friendly vegetarian diet.

Balanced Plant-Based Proteins:

1. Nutritionists emphasize the importance of incorporating a variety of plant-based proteins to ensure a comprehensive amino acid profile. Legumes, such as lentils, chickpeas, and beans, are excellent sources of protein, and when combined with whole grains, nuts, and seeds, they form a complete protein spectrum. Ensuring an adequate intake of protein is essential for overall health and muscle function, especially for individuals with kidney concerns.

Mindful Phosphorus Management:

2. Nutritionists highlight the significance of managing phosphorus intake, as excessive levels can be detrimental to kidney health. While plant-based foods generally contain less absorbable phosphorus than animal products, some high-phosphorus plant foods, such as nuts and seeds, should be consumed in moderation. Cooking techniques like leaching and soaking can help reduce phosphorus content in certain foods, supporting kidney wellness.

Calcium-Rich Plant Sources:

3. Maintaining optimal calcium levels is crucial for bone health, and nutritionists advise individuals to explore plant-based calcium sources. Dark leafy greens like kale and bok choy, fortified plant milks, and tofu made with calcium sulfate are excellent alternatives. Ensuring an adequate intake of calcium while being mindful of phosphorus levels contributes to a balanced kidney-friendly vegetarian diet.

Strategic Potassium Control:

4. Nutritionists stress the importance of managing potassium levels, especially for individuals with kidney issues. While many plant-based foods are high in potassium, including fruits, vegetables, and legumes, portion control and strategic food choices can help regulate potassium intake. Cooking methods, such as boiling or leaching, can further assist in reducing potassium content in certain foods.

Fluid Balance and Hydration:

5. Nutritionists emphasize the significance of maintaining proper fluid balance for kidney health. Adequate hydration supports kidney function and helps flush out waste products. Water, herbal teas, and low-sugar beverages are recommended choices. Monitoring fluid intake becomes essential, especially for individuals with kidney concerns who may need to limit fluid consumption based on their specific health requirements.

Individualized Nutrient Needs:

6. Nutritionists underscore the importance of individualized nutrition plans tailored to specific health needs and preferences. Each person's nutritional requirements vary, and factors such as age, gender, activity level, and overall health should be considered. Consulting with a registered dietitian allows individuals to receive personalized guidance on crafting a kidney-friendly vegetarian diet that aligns with their unique nutritional needs.

Vitamin D and Sun Exposure:

7. Ensuring adequate vitamin D levels is crucial for kidney health, as it plays a role in calcium absorption. Nutritionists recommend incorporating vitamin D-rich foods like fortified plant milks and cereals or considering vitamin D supplements if necessary. Additionally, moderate sun exposure contributes to natural vitamin D synthesis, supporting overall bone and kidney wellness.

Mindful Sodium Consumption:

8. Nutritionists emphasize the importance of mindful sodium control, as excessive salt intake can contribute to hypertension and negatively impact kidney function. Choosing fresh, whole foods and using herbs and spices for flavoring instead of salt are practical strategies. Reading food labels helps identify hidden sources of sodium in processed and packaged vegetarian products.

Gradual Dietary Changes:

9. Nutritionists advocate for gradual dietary changes, especially for those transitioning to a vegetarian lifestyle. Slowly introducing new foods and experimenting with different recipes allows individuals to adapt to the dietary shift while monitoring how their bodies respond. This approach promotes long-term adherence to a kidney-friendly vegetarian diet.

Regular Monitoring and Adjustments:

10. Nutritionists emphasize the importance of regular monitoring of kidney function through medical check-ups and blood tests. Adjustments to the diet may be necessary based on individual health changes and evolving nutritional needs. Nutritionists work collaboratively with healthcare providers to ensure that dietary recommendations align with overall health goals.

In conclusion, insights from nutritionists play a pivotal role in guiding individuals toward a kidney-friendly vegetarian diet. By focusing on balanced plant-based proteins, strategic nutrient management, individualized nutrition plans, and gradual dietary changes, individuals can embrace a vegetarian lifestyle while supporting optimal kidney health. Nutritionists provide valuable expertise in navigating the complexities of dietary choices, empowering individuals to make informed decisions that promote both their vegetarian principles and renal wellness.

- Answering Common Questions

*1. **Q: Can I get enough protein from a vegetarian diet to support kidney health?**

A: Absolutely. While animal products are common protein sources, a well-planned vegetarian diet can provide ample protein. Legumes, tofu, tempeh, nuts, and seeds are rich in protein and can be combined to ensure a complete amino acid profile, supporting kidney health without overloading on phosphorus.

2. Q: Are plant-based proteins as good as animal-based proteins for kidney health?

A: Yes. Plant-based proteins offer numerous health benefits and can be favorable for kidney health. They tend to be lower in phosphorus, which is crucial for those with kidney concerns. Legumes, grains, and plant-based protein products can serve as excellent alternatives to animal proteins while supporting overall well-being.

3. Q: How do I manage phosphorus intake in a vegetarian diet?

A: Focus on moderation and mindful choices. While some plant foods contain phosphorus, it's about balancing the intake. Limit high-phosphorus foods like nuts and seeds, and consider cooking methods that reduce phosphorus, such as leaching or boiling vegetables. Regular monitoring and consulting with a dietitian can help manage phosphorus levels effectively.

4. Q: Can I still enjoy dairy on a kidney-friendly vegetarian diet?

A: Yes, in moderation. Dairy products are good sources of calcium, but they can be high in phosphorus. Opt for lower-phosphorus dairy options or explore plant-based alternatives like almond or rice milk fortified with calcium. Again, moderation is key to strike the right balance.

5. Q: Are there vegetarian sources of calcium for bone health?

A: Absolutely. Dark leafy greens like kale and bok choy, fortified plant milks, and tofu made with calcium sulfate are excellent sources of plant-based calcium. Including these foods in your diet ensures that you meet your calcium needs without compromising kidney health.

6. Q: How can I control potassium intake on a vegetarian diet?

A: Be mindful of high-potassium foods like bananas, oranges, and potatoes. Portion control is essential, and cooking techniques like boiling or leaching can help reduce potassium content. Including a variety of fruits and vegetables while monitoring portions allows you to enjoy a diverse diet without exceeding potassium limits.

7. Q: Is a vegetarian diet suitable for individuals with kidney concerns?

A: Yes, with proper planning. A well-structured vegetarian diet can be suitable for kidney health. It involves choosing the right mix of plant-based proteins, managing phosphorus and potassium levels, and staying hydrated. Consulting with a dietitian ensures that dietary choices align with individual health needs.

8. Q: Can I enjoy vegetarian snacks while following a kidney-friendly diet?

A: Certainly. Opt for kidney-friendly snacks like air-popped popcorn, raw vegetables with hummus, or a small serving of mixed nuts. Reading labels to identify hidden phosphorus or sodium in packaged snacks is essential. Balancing taste and nutrition is achievable with mindful snack choices.

9. Q: How can I add flavor to my meals without using too much salt?

A: Get creative with herbs, spices, and citrus flavors. Fresh herbs like basil, cilantro, and mint, along with spices such as cumin, coriander, and turmeric, can add depth and flavor to your dishes without relying on excessive salt. Experimenting with different combinations enhances the taste of kidney-friendly meals.

10. Q: Can I still enjoy international cuisines on a kidney-friendly vegetarian diet?

A: Absolutely. Many international cuisines offer a variety of plant-based options. For example, Mediterranean cuisine includes dishes like lentil soups and grilled vegetables, and Asian cuisine often features tofu and vegetable stir-fries. Exploring diverse cuisines ensures that you can enjoy flavorful meals while adhering to kidney-friendly guidelines.

11. Q: How do I ensure I'm getting enough vitamins and minerals on a vegetarian diet?

A: Variety is key. Including a diverse range of fruits, vegetables, whole grains, nuts, and seeds ensures you receive a spectrum of essential nutrients. If there are concerns about specific nutrients, consulting with a dietitian can help create a personalized plan to address individual nutritional needs.

12. Q: Can I incorporate plant-based protein powders into my diet for additional protein?

A: Yes, with caution. Plant-based protein powders, such as pea or hemp protein, can be added to smoothies or recipes. However, it's crucial to read labels, choose products with lower phosphorus content, and ensure they align with individual dietary restrictions. Moderation is key to prevent excessive nutrient intake.

In conclusion, adopting a kidney-friendly vegetarian diet involves careful consideration of nutrient intake, balancing protein sources, and making informed choices. With proper planning, moderation, and guidance from healthcare professionals or dietitians, individuals can enjoy the benefits of a vegetarian lifestyle while supporting kidney health. These answers aim to dispel common concerns and provide insights for those navigating the intersection of vegetarianism and kidney wellness.

CHAPTER FOURTEEN

KIDNEY-FRIENDLY DESSERTS

- Berry Parfait

Ingredients:

- 1 cup of mixed berries (such as blueberries, strawberries, and raspberries)
- 1 cup of low-fat or non-fat Greek yogurt
- 1/2 cup of granola (choose a low-phosphorus option)
- One tablespoon of maple syrup or honey, if preferred
- Fresh mint leaves for garnish

Instructions:

Prepare the Berries:

1. Start by washing and chopping the berries. If you're using strawberries, hull and slice them into bite-sized pieces. Berries are not only delicious but also rich in antioxidants, providing a burst of flavor and nutrition to your parfait.

Select Kidney-Friendly Granola:

2. Choose a granola with lower phosphorus content, as excessive phosphorus can be detrimental to kidney health. Look for options that use whole grains and nuts without added phosphorus-based additives. Alternatively, you can make your own granola at home using kidney-friendly ingredients.

Opt for Low-Fat Greek Yogurt:

3. Greek yogurt is an excellent
    source of protein and calcium,
    supporting overall health and
    kidney function. Choose low-fat or
    non-fat varieties to manage fat
    intake. The creaminess of Greek
    yogurt adds a satisfying texture to
    the parfait while contributing
    essential nutrients.

Layering the Parfait:

4. Begin assembling the parfait by layering the ingredients. In a glass or bowl, start with a spoonful of Greek yogurt at the bottom. Add a layer of mixed berries, followed by a sprinkle of Up till the glass's top, keep layering the layers on. colorful layers not only look appealing but also provide a variety of flavors and textures.

Drizzle with Honey or Maple Syrup (Optional):

5. If you desire a touch of sweetness, drizzle a small amount of honey or maple syrup over the top. Keep in mind that excessive sugar intake should be avoided, so use this option sparingly or skip it altogether. The natural sweetness from the berries may be sufficient to satisfy your taste buds.

Garnish with Fresh Mint:

6. Add a finishing touch to your berry parfait by garnishing it with fresh mint leaves. Not only does mint enhance the visual appeal, but it also contributes a refreshing flavor that complements the sweetness of the berries.

Effect on the Body:

Rich in Antioxidants:

1. Berries are packed with antioxidants, such as anthocyanins and vitamin C, which help combat oxidative stress and inflammation. These properties are beneficial for overall health and may contribute to kidney wellness.

Protein and Calcium for Kidney Health:

2. Greek yogurt serves as an excellent source of protein and calcium. Protein is essential for muscle function, and calcium is crucial for bone health. Incorporating these nutrients in a kidney-friendly dessert supports overall well-being.

Moderate Phosphorus Content:

3. By selecting a low-phosphorus granola and being mindful of ingredient choices, this berry parfait helps manage phosphorus intake. Excessive phosphorus can be challenging for individuals with kidney concerns, so it's important to opt for kidney-friendly alternatives.

Hydration from Berries:

4. Because berries contain a lot of water, they help you stay hydrated. Maintaining adequate fluid balance is crucial for kidney health, and incorporating hydrating foods like berries is a delicious way to support this balance.

Customizable and Adaptable:

5. The beauty of a berry parfait lies in its adaptability. You can customize the ingredients based on your preferences and dietary restrictions. Experiment with different berries, granola options, or even alternative yogurt choices to suit your individual needs.

In conclusion, this kidney-friendly berry parfait offers a delightful combination of flavors, textures, and nutrients. It's a satisfying dessert that not only caters to your sweet cravings but also supports overall kidney health. By making mindful ingredient choices and embracing the natural goodness of berries, you can indulge in a delicious treat that aligns with your dietary goals.

- Baked Apple with Cinnamon

Baked apples with cinnamon make for a delightful and kidney-friendly dessert that not only satisfies your sweet tooth but also aligns with dietary considerations for kidney health. This dessert is not only delicious but also incorporates ingredients that are mindful of kidney function.

Ingredients:

1. Apples: Choose firm, fresh apples like Granny Smith or Honeycrisp. These varieties hold up well during baking.
2. Cinnamon: Ground cinnamon adds warmth and a sweet-spicy flavor without the need for excessive sugar.
3. Sweetener: Consider using a kidney-friendly sweetener such as erythritol or monk fruit sweetener to reduce sugar content.
4. Nuts (optional): Chopped almonds or walnuts can add a satisfying crunch and additional nutritional value.

5. Vanilla Extract: A small amount of vanilla extract enhances the overall flavor without compromising kidney health.
6. Butter or Margarine: Use a kidney-friendly butter substitute or margarine to keep saturated fat in check.

Instructions:

1. Preheat the Oven: Set your oven to 375°F (190°C) to ensure it's adequately heated before placing the apples inside.
2. Prepare the Apples: Wash and core the apples, leaving the bottom intact to create a well for the filling. Removing the seeds and excess core helps make room for the delicious stuffing.
3. Mix the Filling: In a bowl, combine cinnamon, sweetener, and a splash of vanilla extract. Adjust the sweetness according to your taste and dietary requirements. If you're adding nuts, mix them into the cinnamon-sweetener mixture.

4. Stuff the Apples: Spoon the
    cinnamon-sweetener mixture into the
    well of each apple. Ensure an even
    distribution of the filling for consistent
    flavor.
5. Top with Butter or Margarine: Place a
    small amount of kidney-friendly butter or
    margarine on top of each stuffed apple.
    This adds a rich, buttery flavor while
    keeping saturated fat levels in check.
6. Bake to Perfection: Arrange the stuffed
    apples in a baking dish and bake in the
    preheated oven for approximately 25-30
    minutes or until the apples are tender.
    Baking time may vary based on the size
    and variety of apples, so keep an eye on
    them.
7. Serve Warm: Once baked, let the apples
    cool slightly before serving. The warmth
    of the baked apples, combined with the
    aromatic cinnamon, creates a
    comforting and inviting dessert.

This kidney-friendly baked apple with cinnamon dessert is a wholesome treat that balances sweetness and nutrition. It provides a satisfying alternative to traditional desserts that may be high in phosphorus, potassium, and sodium, which can be detrimental to kidney health. Enjoy this delightful dessert without compromising on flavor or your well-being.

CHAPTER FIFTEEN

CELEBRATING SPECIAL OCCASION

- ○ Kidney-Friendly Holiday Recipes

The holiday season often brings with it a plethora of rich and indulgent dishes, but for individuals with kidney health concerns, navigating festive feasts can be a challenge. However, with a bit of creativity and mindfulness, it's entirely possible to enjoy delicious, kidney-friendly holiday recipes that cater to dietary restrictions while preserving the joy of the season.

1. Herb-Roasted Turkey Breast:
A centerpiece of many holiday meals, turkey can be prepared in a kidney-friendly way by opting for a lean turkey breast. Season it with a mix of

kidney-safe herbs like rosemary, thyme, and sage, along with garlic and a dash of olive oil. Roast until the skin is golden and the meat is cooked to perfection. This dish provides a protein-rich option without the excess sodium often found in pre-packaged seasonings.

2. Mashed Cauliflower:
Swap traditional mashed potatoes, which can be high in potassium, with mashed cauliflower. Boil cauliflower until tender, then mash it with a bit of low-sodium chicken broth, garlic, and a touch of kidney-friendly butter substitute. The result is a creamy and flavorful alternative that's lower in potassium.

3. Green Bean Almondine:
Green beans are a kidney-friendly vegetable choice. Sauté them with sliced almonds, a hint of lemon juice, and a touch of olive oil. This side dish is not only kidney-friendly but also adds a burst of color to your holiday spread.

4. Quinoa and Cranberry Salad:

Create a nutrient-packed salad by combining cooked quinoa, dried cranberries, chopped parsley, and a light vinaigrette made with kidney-friendly ingredients like olive oil and lemon juice. This dish is a refreshing and satisfying addition to your holiday table.

5. Baked Salmon with Dill Sauce:

Salmon is an excellent source of omega-3 fatty acids and a kidney-friendly protein option. Bake salmon fillets with a sprinkle of dill and a touch of lemon. Serve with a homemade dill sauce made with low-fat sour cream or a kidney-friendly yogurt alternative.

6. Butternut Squash Soup:

Butternut squash, when pureed into a soup, delivers a velvety texture and rich flavor. Season it with nutmeg, cinnamon, and a touch of low-sodium vegetable broth. This soup is not only kidney-friendly but also a comforting starter for your holiday meal.

7. Roasted Brussels Sprouts with Bacon (Optional):

Brussels sprouts are a low-potassium vegetable that can be roasted to perfection. Add a savory twist by including small amounts of lean bacon for flavor. Roasting enhances the natural sweetness of Brussels sprouts while creating a satisfying side dish.

8. Kidney-Friendly Stuffing:

Prepare stuffing using whole-grain bread, low-sodium chicken broth, and a medley of kidney-friendly herbs. Add chopped celery, onions, and a sprinkle of poultry seasoning for a delicious stuffing that aligns with kidney health guidelines.

9. Cranberry Sorbet:

For a kidney-friendly dessert option, consider making cranberry sorbet. Blend cranberries with water, a touch of sweetener, and a squeeze of lemon . Mixture should be frozen until sorbet-like consistency is achieved. This refreshing treat is a festive way to end your holiday meal.

10. Baked Apples with Cinnamon (as previously mentioned):
Round out your holiday feast with a kidney-friendly dessert like baked apples with cinnamon. It's a warm and comforting treat that satisfies your sweet cravings without compromising kidney health.

Conclusion:
Celebrating the holidays with kidney health in mind doesn't mean sacrificing flavor or festive traditions. By choosing kidney-friendly ingredients and adapting traditional recipes, you can create a holiday spread that is both delicious and supportive of renal well-being. Remember to consult with a healthcare professional or a dietitian to tailor these recipes to your specific dietary needs and restrictions. Embrace the joy of the season while

taking care of your kidneys with these thoughtfully crafted holiday recipes.

○ Tips for Celebrating with Dietary Restrictions

A kidney-friendly vegetarian diet, requires a thoughtful approach to ensure both enjoyment and adherence to health guidelines. Here are some tips to make festivities flavorful and kidney-conscious while embracing a vegetarian lifestyle.

1. Understand Your Dietary Needs:
Before planning any celebration, it's crucial to have a clear understanding of your dietary needs and restrictions. Consult with a healthcare professional or a registered dietitian to determine specific guidelines based on your kidney health. This guarantees that the foods you eat are in line with your general health.

2. Explore Plant-Based Proteins:

Embrace a variety of plant-based proteins to meet your nutritional requirements without overloading on potassium and phosphorus.For vegans, legumes including black beans, chickpeas, and lentils are great sources of protein.Tofu and tempeh are also kidney-friendly options that can be incorporated into various dishes.

3. Opt for Whole Grains:

For more fiber and minerals, go for whole grains rather than processed grains.Brown rice, quinoa, bulgur, and whole wheat products are good choices. These grains contribute to a well-rounded vegetarian diet while offering essential nutrients without compromising kidney health.

4. Mindful Meal Planning:

Plan your meals ahead of time, considering your dietary restrictions. Include a balance of vegetables, fruits, grains, and plant-based proteins in your daily intake. This planning helps you create diverse and satisfying meals that meet your nutritional needs while keeping potassium and phosphorus levels in check.

5. Limit High-Potassium Foods:
While many plant-based foods are rich in potassium, it's essential to moderate your intake. Potatoes, tomatoes, and certain fruits like bananas and oranges are high in potassium. Control portions and consider alternative ingredients to reduce potassium levels in your meals.

6. Experiment with Low-Potassium Vegetables:
Incorporate low-potassium vegetables into your diet to maintain variety and nutritional balance. Bell peppers, cabbage, cauliflower, and zucchini are examples of vegetables that are lower in potassium. Experiment with different cooking methods to keep your meals exciting and flavorful.

7. Homemade Sauces and Dressings:

Create kidney-friendly sauces and dressings at home to control sodium and phosphorus content. Opt for herbs, spices, and vinegar to add flavor without comprom sing your dietary restrictions. This allows you to enjoy tasty, homemade dishes without the excess salt often found in store-bought condiments.

8. Stay Hydrated:
Proper hydration is crucial for kidney health. Make sure you stay hydrated throughout the day by drinking enough water.If you're attending a celebration, bring your own water or choose low-potassium beverages to stay hydrated without overloading on kidney-stressing elements.

9. Communicate Dietary Needs:
When attending gatherings or celebrations, don't hesitate to communicate your dietary needs to the host or chef. Many people are accommodating and will appreciate knowing in advance if there are

specific dietary considerations. This helps ensure there are suitable options available for you to enjoy.

10. Potluck Contribution:

Consider contributing a kidney-friendly vegetarian dish to potluck-style gatherings. This not only guarantees you have a safe option to enjoy but also introduces others to delicious and health-conscious vegetarian recipes. Share your culinary creations, sparking interest in kidney-friendly eating among friends and family.

11. Mindful Snacking:

Choose kidney-friendly snacks to curb between-meal cravings. Nuts and seeds, while generally healthy, can be high in phosphorus, so opt for lower-phosphorus options like air-popped popcorn or vegetable sticks with a kidney-friendly dip.

12. Dessert Alternatives:

Satisfy your sweet tooth with kidney-friendly dessert alternatives. Fruit sorbets, like the cranberry sorbet mentioned earlier, or a refreshing fruit salad, can provide a sweet ending to a meal without compromising your dietary restrictions.

13. Educate Yourself and Others:
Stay informed about kidney-friendly vegetarian options and share your knowledge with others. By educating friends and family about your dietary needs, you create a supportive environment that allows everyone to enjoy the celebration together.

Conclusion:

Celebrating with dietary restrictions as a kidney-friendly vegetarian requires a combination of preparation, communication, and creativity. By understanding your specific dietary needs, exploring diverse plant-based options, and planning meals mindfully, you can navigate festivities with confidence. Remember that celebrations are about joy, connection, and delicious food, and with thoughtful choices, you can enjoy the best of both worlds – a flavorful, kidney-conscious vegetarian lifestyle and the joyous spirit of celebrations.

CONCLUSION

Embracing a kidney-friendly lifestyle is not just a culinary journey; it's a commitment to your well-being, a pledge to nurture your body with the wholesome goodness of kidney-friendly vegetarian choices. As we conclude this culinary adventure tailored for beginners, let's reflect on the transformative power of our choices and the impact they can have on our kidney health.

In the tapestry of our lives, food is the vibrant thread that weaves through every moment. It holds the potential to either fortify or undermine our health, especially when it comes to our kidneys. The recipes shared in this cookbook are not mere instructions; they are invitations to embrace a lifestyle that cherishes and supports the incredible work our kidneys do for us.

Our journey began with the understanding that a kidney-friendly diet doesn't mean sacrificing flavor or variety. Instead, it opens up a world of culinary exploration where every ingredient serves a purpose—nourishing our bodies while tantalizing our taste buds. We learned that plant-based foods can be powerful allies in promoting kidney health, offering a symphony of textures and tastes that elevate our meals to a new level.

In the pages preceding this conclusion, we've discovered the magic of incorporating kidney-friendly superfoods into our daily meals. From the vibrant crunch of leafy greens to the satisfying richness of plant-based proteins, every recipe is a celebration of balance. We've seen how mindful choices in ingredients can make a significant difference in supporting kidney function and overall well-being.

But this cookbook is more than just a collection of recipes; it's a guide to a kidney-friendly lifestyle. As we close this chapter, let's consider a few essential principles that can help solidify this commitment in our daily lives.

1. Hydration is Key:

Remember to stay adequately hydrated. Water is a gentle yet potent ally for kidney health. It helps flush out toxins and ensures that our kidneys can efficiently perform their vital functions. Make it a habit to keep a water bottle close by, a constant reminder of your commitment to hydration.

2. Mindful Moderation:

While the recipes provided are kidney-friendly, moderation remains a cornerstone of a healthy lifestyle. Pay attention to portion sizes, savoring each bite mindfully. By doing so, you not only enjoy your meals more fully but also allow your body to process nutrients optimally.

3. Regular Exercise:

Pair your newfound culinary skills with regular physical activity. Exercise is a catalyst for overall well-being, and it complements the benefits of a kidney-friendly diet. Whether it's a brisk walk, yoga, or any activity you enjoy, incorporating movement into your routine enhances the holistic approach to kidney health.

4. Routine Check-ups:

Lastly, maintain regular check-ups with your healthcare provider. Monitoring your kidney function ensures early detection of any potential issues, allowing for timely intervention. Your commitment to a kidney-friendly lifestyle goes hand in hand with proactive healthcare.

As you embark on this journey towards a kidney-friendly lifestyle, remember that every meal is an opportunity to nourish not just your body but also your spirit. Your culinary choices are a form of self-care, a daily affirmation of your commitment to a healthier and more vibrant life.

In conclusion, let this cookbook be your companion on the path to kidney-friendly living. May these recipes inspire you to create nourishing, flavorful meals that elevate your well-being. Embrace this lifestyle not as a restrictive diet but as a celebration of the incredible resilience and adaptability of the human body.

The power to transform your health lies in your hands, quite literally, as you chop, sauté, and savor each ingredient. So, let's raise our utensils in a toast to embracing a kidney-friendly lifestyle—one delicious and healthful meal at a time. Your journey has just begun, and the possibilities for a vibrant, kidney-friendly life are as expansive as your imagination allows.

Here's to your health, vitality, and the joy of savoring every moment on this nourishing path. Cheers to a kidney-friendly life!

www.ingramcontent.com/pod-product-compliance
Lightning Source LLC
Chambersburg PA
CBHW070923260726
48661CB00003B/805